Secret Shaolin Formulas for the Treatment of External Injury

Chapter Number Ten of
Shao Lin Si Mi Fang Ji Jin
Highlights of Shaolin Monastery's Secret Prescriptions

Orally Transmitted by
PATRIARCH DE CHAN

Recorded & Arranged by
MONK DE QIAN

Translated by
ZHANG TING-LIANG
&
BOB FLAWS

Second Edition Revised and Edited by
BOB FLAWS

BLUE POPPY PRESS

Published by:

**BLUE POPPY PRESS
1775 LINDEN AVE.
BOULDER, CO 80304**

SECOND EDITION, JANUARY 1995

ISBN 0-936185-08-2 LC #94-78715

COPYRIGHT 1995 © BLUE POPPY PRESS

All rights reserved. No part of this book may be reproduced, stored in a retrieval system, or transcribed in any form or by any means, electronic, mechanical, photocopy, recording, or any other means, without the prior written permission of the publisher.

The information in this book is given in good faith. However, the translators and the publisher cannot be held responsible for any error or omission. Nor can they be held in any way responsible for treatment given on the basis of information contained in this book. The publishers make this information available to English language readers for scholarly and research purposes only.

The publishers do not advocate nor endorse self-medication by laypersons. Chinese medicine is a professional medicine. Laypersons interested in availing themselves of the treatments described in this book should seek out a qualified professional practitioner of Chinese medicine.

COMP Designation: Original work and functionally translated compilation

Printed at Westview Press, Boulder, CO on acid free, recycled paper.
Cover printed at C & M Press, Denver, CO
Cover Calligraphy by Zhang Ting-liang

10 9 8 7 6 5 4 3

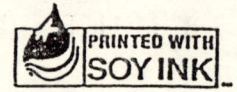

朱店神传千秋
今朝更敬爱人民

当山岩德禅
一九八四年青

Translator's Preface to the Second Blue Poppy Edition

The following book is the second, revised edition of a translation of the first ten chapters of Book One of *Shao Lin Si Mi Fang Ji Jin (Highlights of the Shaolin Monastery's Secret Formulas)* published by the Henan Science & Technology Press in 1986. This translation was originally done by Zhang Ting-liang and myself in 1987, and I did the revised translation for this edition in 1994. Based on the definitions of the Council of Oriental Medical Publishers (COMP), this is a connotative translation using a standard translational terminology in terms of the Chinese medical terms. In addition, we have moved the biography of De Chan, the author, which appears as an appendix in the Chinese original, to the front of the book.

The original text was orally transmitted by the 31st Patriarch of the Shaolin Monastery, the Abbot De Chan, to the monk De Qian. De Qian spent three years receiving this transmission. He then recorded, arranged, and annotated these prescriptions. De Chan was 77 years old at the time of this transmission. As a monk doctor he was well versed in the martial arts and in the treatment of trauma and had over 60 years of personal clinical experience. Book One's heading is *Shao Lin Si Die Da Sun Shang Fang* which means *Shaolin Monastery Fall & Strike Injury Formulas*.

This book is an important addition to the English literature on Chinese medicine for several reasons. First, it is of practical value to all clinicians practicing Chinese medicine. In it are found the indications, ingredients, methods of preparation, dosages, and commentary of 268 previously untranslated "secret" formulas for the treatment of *shang ke* (traumatology) and *die da* (injury due to fall and strike).

Secondly, this book is an example of a Buddhist lineage of Chinese medicine. Although it has been arranged according to the format of many other contemporary Traditional Chinese Medicine texts, it clearly records and presents a non-TCM style of Chinese medicine. So-called Traditional Chinese Medicine, or TCM, is the government-approved, essentially Confucian style of Chinese medicine dominant in the People's Republic of China today. In the original Chinese introduction to this book, the Abbot De Chan is described as a practitioner of *seng yi* or Buddhist monk medicine as opposed to *zhong yi*, Chinese medicine or TCM. There is also a reference to *si yuan seng yi* or "the monastic schools of Buddhist medicine," and the commentaries on many of the prescriptions give ample evidence of generations of monk doctors. Although the text of this book is bereft of any of the spiritual practices and perspectives that one might expect accompanying the practice of Buddhist medicine, still this book is a link to a historically verifiable but nonetheless different style of Chinese medicine than TCM.

Thirdly, this book contains treatments for problems caused by improper *qi gong* and *wu shu* training. Many Western martial artists and students of *qi gong* and *tai ji quan* will benefit by access to these treatments. Also, the existence of such treatments underscores the fact that such training should be approached with care and understanding since improper training may definitely lead to serious physical and mental problems.

In 1987 when Blue Poppy Press published its first edition of this translation, the text was composed on an electronic typewriter. When this edition was allowed to go out of print in 1992, it was because of three reasons. First, the physical design and production of this book

Translator's Preface

was far below Blue Poppy's current standard. Secondly, the medicinal identifications were given in Latin only without Pinyin. Ever since its initial publication, our readers have complained about the lack of Pinyin, making the identification and especially the purchase of the ingredients described herein difficult. And third, since 1987, Blue Poppy Press has adopted Nigel Wiseman's translational terminology as our standard, and, therefore, the terms in our original translation were not consistent with other, more recent Blue Poppy publications. However, there never seemed to be the time to go back and put in those Pinyin identifications, update the terminology, and redesign the book. Finally, after accumulating more than 100 names and addresses of potential customers waiting for a reissue, M. Robert Rinchart of S.A.T.A.S. in Belgium prevailed upon me to *make* the time to do the necessary corrections and additions.

In order to make this book as clinically useful as possible, we have added a few footnotes to the original text, particularly in reference to the preparation and processing of various ingredients. Knowledge of such preparation techniques was presupposed by the author and is part of basic Chinese medical training. Information in the footnotes concerning herbal preparation is based on *Xin Bian Zhong Yao Pao Zhi Fa (A New Compendium of Processing Methods for Chinese Medicinals)* by Ma Zing-ning, Shanxi Science & Technology Press, 1984, and on my lecture notes from and clinical practice at the Shanghai College of Traditional Chinese Medicine.

The identifications of medicinals in this book are based on Bensky & Gamble's *Chinese Herbal Medicine: Materia Medica*; Hong-yen Hsu's *Oriental Materia Medica: A Concise Guide;* Stuart & Reid's *Chinese Materia Medica*; and the *Zhong Yao Da Ci Dian (The Encyclopedia of Chinese Medicinals)* published by the Shanghai Science & Technology Press. The few ingredients we have not been able to identify have been given in Pinyin with their Chinese characters following in parentheses. Some ingredients which are

Secret Shaolin Formulas

common foods or substances in Chinese culture we have translated as simply as possible, such as monkey bones, bear's palms, and day lily buds. In preparing this revised edition, we have corrected a number of misidentified medicinals, identified a number of medicinals we failed to identify in the first edition, and added some medicinals which were inadvertently left out of the first edition. Thus we believe the medicinal identifications in this edition are far superior to the previous version.

Acupuncture point nomenclature as it appears in this book is based on the World Health Organization's *Proposed Standard International Acupuncture Nomenclature* with the following differences: First, we give the Pinyin romanization of the name first followed by channel abbreviation and number in parentheses. Secondly, we have separated each Pinyin syllable. Just as one does not write Newyork or Northdakota, we feel it is incorrect in English to write *Sibai*. This means Four Whites and is a proper name made up of two distinct words. For instance, the translator does not write his name Robertsuttonflaws. And third, in terms of the abbreviations for channel identifications, we use Lu for WHO's LU, St for ST, Sp for SP, Ht for HT, Per for PC, TH for TE, Bl for BL, and Liv for LR.

The headings and organization of each prescription appear as they do in the original. There is a certain amount of inconsistency as might be expected from an oral transmission. The Commentary sections appended to many of the prescriptions are from the Chinese original as are those headed **Note**. Typically, the commentaries contain historical anecdotes regarding the prescription in question. Whereas the notes contain more miscellaneous information, such as contraindications and explanations of obscure or technical terms. We have mostly limited our comments to the footnotes. In a few cases, we have been able to identify and rectify typographical errors in the Chinese original.

Translator's Preface

The dosages of the majority of ingredients are given in metric notation. G stands for grams. Ml stands for milliliters. One *ji* usually means one day's dose. The word *ji* literally means prescription or formula. However, when used as a description of amounts of a formula to be taken, 1 *ji* means one packet of the stated formula.

Often the text does not specify how much water to use in the decoction of the ingredients nor how many times per day to take the medicine or when. Unless otherwise indicated, I suggest the following guidelines. Place one dose or packet of herbs in a lidded pot. Cover with water or other specified combination of liquids so that 1-2 fingerwidths of liquid extend over the top of the herbs. Allow the herbs to soak in this liquid for 1 hour. Then bring the liquid to a boil and cook over moderate heat for approximately 30 minutes. Formulas containing supplementing medicinals should be cooked for closer to an hour. Stones and bones should be decocted in advance for 1 hour before adding the other pre-soaked ingredients. Some flowers and leaves which are aromatic should be added at the end to steep, such as Flos Chrysanthemi Morifolii (*Ju Hua*). Fragrant medicinals for rectifying the qi, such as Radix Saussureae Seu Vladimiriae (*Mu Xiang*), should not be cooked for more than 7 minutes, nor should cold medicinals, such as Rhizoma Coptidis Chinensis (*Huang Lian*). Gelatins should be dissolved and taken separately. Likewise, powdered Radix Pseudoginseng (*Tian Qi* or *San Qi*) and some mineral powders, such as Cinnabar (*Zhu Sha*) and Mirabilitum (*Mang Xiao*), should also be taken separately chased down with warm water. Fresh Rhizoma Zingiberis (*Sheng Jiang*) should be added during the last 5 minutes of decoction and should only be simmered gently.

Strain off the liquid and take 1 teacup of liquid (soup, juice, tea, or whatever you care to call it). Take either 1 hour before or 2 hours after meals. If formulas are meant to go to the lower half of the body, they should be taken before meals. If they are meant to affect the upper half of the body, take after meals. If herbs are harsh or difficult

ix

to digest, take soon after a meal to protect the stomach qi. Also digestant formulas should be taken soon after meals in order to aid digestion and absorption of nutrients. A second cup of liquid can be obtained by adding more water or other liquid to the herbs and decocting them again as above. In this case, they need not be soaked again. Herbs which should be steeped, powders taken separately, and gelatins dissolved separately should be added fresh. Likewise, fresh ginger should be added again during the last 5 minutes of cooking. Strain off the liquid and take the second cup later the same day.

As mentioned above, the translational terminology used in preparing this revised edition is based on Nigel Wiseman's *Glossary of Chinese Medical Terms and Acupuncture Points*, Paradigm Publications, Brookline, MA.

Bob Flaws
August 1994

Abbot De Chan's Biography

Abbot De Chan's family name was Liu and his given names were Er-he. He was born in Zuo Zhuang village, Cheng Guan Zheng in Feng Deng County, Henan Province, in 1907. Because of the death of his father during his youth and several years of natural calamities, (seeing the futility of samsaric existence, De Chan) was forced to leave his family (and the householder's life) and entered Shaolin Monastery on Mt. Song in 1916 (the 5th year of the Chinese Republic). There he became the student of Monk Su Guang. As a novice, he was required to do many jobs about the monastery. Because of his respect for the senior monks and his diligent studies, he soon became loved by all. (Therefore,) he was sent to the monastery school the following year and graduated from Shaolin Middle School in 1920.

Because of his perseverance and devotion, Zhen Jun, De Chan's senior teacher, recommended that he be sent to study Buddhist medicine from a well-known monk doctor at Huang Wan Monastery, Ji Xue, in 1921. He read the medical classics earnestly and practiced hard. Due to his painstaking effort, De Chan graduated with excellent academic score in 1924 and then returned to the Shaolin Monastery. In May, De Chan became the head of Hui San Monastery, a branch monastery of Shaolin. He returned to the Shaolin Monastery as an ordinary monk and doctor in 1927.

In 1928, Shi You-san, a Guo Min Dang (KMT) military officer was ordered to burn down the Shaolin Monastery. Some of the monks fled as a consequence, but De Chan organized the martial monks to fight the Guo Min Dang soldiers and to protect the property of the monastery.

After Liberation, De Chan became a member of the county health association. He collected herbs up on the mountain by himself and made them into pills, elixirs, powders, pastes, and liniments for the treatment of a wide variety of diseases for the masses. Because of this, De Chan won the respect and admiration of the people in the seven counties surrounding the monastery for one hundred *li*.

In April 1979, Zhong Dao-cheng, the great monk and Chairman of the Union of Shaolin Martial Arts in Japan, came on pilgrimage to the Shaolin Monastery and paid Abbot De Chan a visit. They had a cordial conversation and from that time maintained a profound friendship. In the spring of that year, a monument with the following inscription was erected in the "Forest of Monuments": "Return of Zhong Dao-cheng, the Japanese great monk." (At that time,) Zhong Dao-cheng asked his daughter, Zhong You-gui, to henceforth call De Chan her adopted father. Since the death of Zhong Dao-cheng, Zhong You-gui, who succeeded her father as Chairperson of the Union, has led a delegation to the monastery every year to call on her adoptive father.

In recent years, Abbot De Chan has received scores of delegations from the United States, Great Britain, West Germany, France, and Singapore and a number of foreign government leaders contributing to the promotion of cultural exchange between China and other countries and friendship among all the peoples of the world.

In 1965, Abbot De Chan was appointed head of the monastery presiding over all its affairs. He became a member of the Buddhist Association of China in November 1982. In January 1982, he was the head of the committee for collecting and collating all the Shaolin martial arts techniques. In December 1982, De Chan was appointed Honorary Chairman of the Shaolin Monastery Association of Feng Deng County. In December of that same year, De Chan was elected First Deputy Chairman of the Buddhist Association of Henan Province, and in April 1984, De Chan became Chairman of the

Buddhist Association of Zheng Zhou municipality in Henan.

From 1981 to 1983, Abbot De Chan organized the disciples both within and without the monastery in systematizing and compiling the *Shao Lin Quan Pu (Shaolin Boxing Manuals)* in 38 volumes and the *Shao Lin Ben Cao (Shaolin Materia Medica)* in 5 volumes.

In 1983, De Chan began transmitting his secret manuscripts and his scores of years of clinical experience to his Buddhist disciples. Having the honor of collecting and collating the secret formulas of the monk doctors of the monastery, I (De Qian) wrote this *Shao Lin Si Mi Fang Ji Jin (Highlights of the Shaolin Monastery's Secret Formulas)*, which is now available to readers, in an attempt to transmit the medical techniques of the monastery and to advance the best of Chinese medicine and health care.

September 1, 1984
Shaolin Monastery

Table of Contents

Translator's Preface to the Second Blue Poppy Edition   v

Abbot De Chan's Biography .... **xi**

Chapter One: Emergency Formulas For Martial Injury   1

    1. Shaolin Recover the Pulse Powder
    2. Shaolin Troop Deployment Powder
    3. Shaolin Precious Jade Powder
    4. First Aid Prescription for Hematemesis Due to Injury to the Precordium
    5. Prescription for the Treatment of Fainting Due to Injury to *Bai Hui* (GV 20)
    6. Shaolin Seizing Life Powder
    7. Two Flavors Recover Life Powder
    8. Treatment of Unstoppable Hematemesis
    9. Recover the Pulse Decoction
    10. Five Treasure Elixir

Chapter Two: Stop Bleeding Formulas **9**

    11. Shaolin Stop Bleeding Powder
    12. Three Treasures Stop Bleeding Powder
    13. Shaolin Metal Injury Powder
    14. Yang Family Spear Wound Powder
    15. Rx for the Treatment of Bleeding Due to Injury of the Nose
    16. Rx for the Treatment of Nose Bleed
    17. Rx for the Treatment of Hematuria Due to Injury of the Lower Abdomen
    18. Rx for the Treatment of Hemafecia Due to Injury of the Lower Abdomen
    19. Rx for the Treatment of Bleeding from the 7 Portals Due to Injury
    20. Rx for the Treatment of Bleeding from the Eye

21. Shaolin Ten Thousand Abilities Stop Bleeding Powder

Chapter Three: Fall, Strike, Bruise & Contusion Formulas . 15

22. Rx for the Treatment of Bruises & Swelling Due to External Injury
23. Rx for the Treatment of Insidious Pain of the Chest & Lateral Costal Area Caused by Hit by Fist
24. Rx for the Treatment of Pain of the Lower Abdomen Due to Hit
25. Rx for the Treatment of Injury to the Sinews Due to Fist or Weapon
26. Technique for the Treatment of Dislocation of the Jaw
27. Rx for the Treatment of Swelling & Pain of the Face Due to Hit Injury
28. Rx for the Treatment of Localized Incessant Pain Due to Hit Injury
29. Rx for the Treatment of Injury to the Sinews Due to Fist & Stick
30. Rx for the Treatment of Bruise & Swelling Due to Injury by Fist
31. Rx for the Treatment of Insidious Pain of the Precordium Due to Strike by Fist
32. Rx for the Treatment of Injury to the Head
33. Rx for the Treatment of Chest Pain Due to Fist Injury
34. Rx for the Treatment of Headache at the Corner of the Forehead Due to Fist Hit
35. Rx for the Treatment of Insidious Pain of the Lower Abdomen Due to Fist Hit
36. Rx for the Treatment of Low Back Pain Due to Injury by Stick
37. Rx for the Treatment of Swelling & Pain of the Nape of the Neck Due to Injury by Stick
38. Rx for the Treatment of Headache of the Forehead Due to Hit by Stick
39. Rx for the Treatment of Swelling & Pain of the Shoulder Due to Hit of Whip
40. Rx for the Treatment of Injury of the Body Due to Hit of Stick & Sudden Fall
41. Rx for the Treatment of Pain in the Right Lateral Costal Area Due to Fist Strike
42. Rx for the Treatment of Pain of the Right Costal Area

43. Rx for the Treatment of Injury Due to Fall because of Unexpected Push
44. Nine Dragon Decoction
45. Rx for the Treatment of Redness & Swelling Due to Injury by Fist or Stick
46. Rx for the Treatment of Skin Rupture in the Area of Injury
47. Rx for the Treatment of Ulcerous Lesions in the Area of Injury
48. Rx for the Treatment of Post Injury Hemorrhagic Dizziness
49. Rx for the Treatment of Failure to Generate New (Tissue) in Enduring Ulcerous Wounds
50. Rx for the Treatment of Greenish Appearance & Discharge of Pus from Affected Area
51. Rx for the Treatment of Injury to the Head by Stick
52. Rx for the Treatment of Neck Hit by Fist
53. Rx for the Treatment of Injury to the Neck Caused by Halberd
54. Shaolin Extract Toxins & Engender Flesh Powder
55. Rx for the Treatment of Injury Due to Falling
56. Rx for the Treatment of Blunt Injury to the Instep
57. Rx for the Treatment of Failure to Recover After Arrow Injury
58. Rx for the Treatment of Shovel Injury to the Shoulder
59. Rx for the Treatment of Injury to the Bone Due to Poisonous Arrow
60. Shaolin Original Brightness Powder
61. Shaolin Red Origin Powder
62. Shaolin Bone Healing Decoction
63. Shaolin Metal Injury Treatment Method
64. Metal Injury Miraculous Recovery Elixir
65. Seven Ingredients Recover & Recuperate Powder
66. Shaolin Pull Out Toxins Plaster
67. Shaolin Expelling Toxins Decoction
68. Shaolin Attack Toxins Powder
69. Injured Sinews Remove the Bone Pills
70. Flying Dragon Life-robbing Elixir
71. Shaolin Seven *Li* Powder
72. Shaolin Strengthen Sinews & Connect the Bones Elixir
73. Soothe the Sinews & Quicken the Network Vessels Decoction
74. Shaolin *Dang Gui* Drink
75. Shaolin Great Strength Pills
76. Shaolin Heroes Pill
77. Shaolin Quicken the Blood Elixir
78. Shaolin Extend the Sinews Elixir
79. Shaolin Nine Tigers Elixir

80. Shaolin Level Wind Elixir
81. Shaolin Eight Immortals Powder
82. Shaolin Three Immortals Powder
83. Shaolin Wintertime Troop Deployment Powder
84. Shaolin Medicinal Thread
85. Shaolin Eight Battle Formations Elixir
86. Five Raw Anesthetics Powder
87. Shaolin Connect the Bones Elixir
88. Connect the Bones Decoction
89. Shaolin Spirit Connecting Powder
90. Rx for the Treatment of *Jin Na Luo* Injury of the Sinews & Bones
91. Five Yellows Powder

Chapter Four: Shaolin Medicinal Wines 59

92. Shaolin Five Fragrances Wine
93. Protect the General Wine
94. Shaolin Live Dragon Wine
95. Long-winded Emperor Assist Training Wine
96. Shaolin Great Supplement Wine
97. Shaolin Abundant Justice Wine

Chapter Five: Shaolin Herbal Plasters 69

98. Toad Skin Plaster
99. Shaolin Return Spring Plaster
100. Shaolin 1,000 Hammers Plaster
101. Shaolin Five Immortals Plaster
102. Shaolin Temple Music Plaster
103. Shaolin White-coated Bodhisattva Plaster
104. Shaolin Medical Ulcer Plaster
105. Five Twigs Plaster
106. Shaolin Three Yellows Plaster
107. Shaolin Toxin-resolving Plaster
108. Shaolin Ten Thousand Respondings Plaster
109. Shaolin Scalding Injury Plaster
110. Shaolin Gentleman's Companion Plaster

Chapter Six: Shaolin Folk & Home Remedies 87

111. Dryland Pipe Tobacco Stop Bleeding Rx
112. Rx to stop Bleeding from Internal or External Injury
113. Rx for the Treatment of Post-trauma Hemafecia & Hematuria

Chapter Seven: Prescriptions For The Treatment Of Injury Due To *Dian Xue* Or Spotting 89

114. Rx for the Treatment of Spotting Injury to *Tan Men* (Liv 14)
115. Rx ... *Xue Qi* (GB 34)
116. Rx ... *Xue Chi* (Sp 10)
117. Rx ... *Qi Kou* (*Bai Lao*) (M-HN-30)
118. Rx ... *Shen Guan* (Ht 7)
119. Rx ... *Ming Gong* (GV 4)
120. Rx ... *Qiao Bun* (Ki 9)
121. Rx ... *Wai Shen* (testes)
122. Rx ... *Wei Gong*
123. Rx ... *Xiao Du Pang* (Sp 15)
124. Rx ... *Feng Guan* (GB 20)
125. Rx ... *Shen Shu* (Bl 23)
126. Rx ... *Feng Wei*
127. Rx ... *Tian Ping* (GV 24)
128. Rx ... *Feng Men* (Bl 12)
129. Rx ... *Bai Hui* (GV 20)
130. Rx ... *Tai Yang* (M-HN-9)
131. Rx ... *Hong Tang*
132. Rx ... *Zhi Shi* (Bl 52)
133. Rx ... *Jian Wo* (LI 15)
134. Rx ... *Ming Mai* (Lu 9)
135. Rx ... *Mai Zong* (Per 6)
136. Rx ... *Tan Tu*
137. Rx ... *Xuan Ji* (CV 21)
138. Rx ... *Suo Xin* (CV 15)
139. Rx ... *Fei Miao* (Ki 27)
140. Rx ... *Wan Xin* (Per 7)
141. Rx ... *Diao Jin*
142. Rx ... *Zhuan Xin* (Bl 15)
143. Rx ... *Fei Shu* (Bl 13)
144. Rx ... *Shi Cang* (CV 10)
145. Rx ... *Xue Chang* (Bl 17)

146. Rx ... *Dan Zhu* (B 19)
147. Rx ... *You Guan* (Ki 21)
148. Rx ... *Tan Ning* (CV 17)
149. Rx ... *Gan Jing*
150. Rx ... *Tian Zong* (SI 11)
151. Rx ... *Shi Jie*
152. Rx ... *Hai Jiao*
153. Rx ... *Qi Shi*
154. Rx ... *Hua Gai*
155. Rx ... *Fei Du* (GB 24)
156. Rx ... *Zheng Qi*
157. Rx ... *Qi Hai* (CV 6)
158. Rx ... *Xue Hai* (Sp 10)
159. Rx ... *Xia Xue Hai*
160. Rx ... *Qi Xue Er Hai*
161. Rx ... *Hei Fu* (CV 13)
162. Rx ... *Huo Fei*
163. Rx ... *Fan Du* (Liv 13)
164. Rx ... *Fu Jie* (Sp 14)
165. Rx ... *Dan Tian*
166. Rx ... *Shui Fen* (CV 9)
167. Rx ... *Qi Ge*
168. Rx ... *Guan Yuan* (CV 4)
169. Rx ... *Xue Hai Men*
170. Rx ... *Qi Ge Men*
171. Rx ... *Xue Nang*
172. Rx ... *Wei Cang*
173. Rx ... *Mei Xin* (*Yin Tang*) (M-HN-3)
174. Rx ... *Qi Men* (Liv 14)
175. Rx ... *Zheng E*
176. Rx ... *Xue Nang He*
177. Rx ... *Da Chang Shu* (Bl 25)
178. Rx ... *Ming Men* (GV 4)
179. Rx ... *Chang Xue* (Bl 18)
180. Rx ... *Xue Zhu* (aorta), *Zhu Ming* (GV 6), *Zan Ming* (GV 16), *Hei Fu Tao Xing* (CV 12), *Gui Yin* (CV 22), *You Hun* (Bl 7)
181. Rx ... Various Points on the Back
182. Rx ... *Hai Di* (Bl 28)
183. Rx ... *Yao Yan* (M-BW-24)
184. Rx ... *Ming Men* (GV 4)
185. Rx ... *Xia Hai Di* (CV 2)
186. Rx ... *He Kou*

187. Rx ... *Yong Quan* (Ki 1)
188. Rx ... *Jing Ming* (Bl 1)
189. Rx ... *Er Men* (TH 21)
190. Rx ... *Nei Guan* (Per 6)
191. Rx ... *Xia Guan* (St 7)

Chapter Eight: Shaolin Herbal Lore 119

192. General Emergency Formula for Spotting (a.k.a. Thirteen Flavors Ruling Formula)
193. Shaolin Toxin-expelling Decoction
194. Modified Thirteen Flavors Rx
195. Shaolin Monastery Secret Transmission Herbal Lore
196. Rx for Effusing & Scattering the Upper Part
197. Rx for Effusing & Scattering the Middle Part
198. Rx for Effusing & Scattering the Lower Part

Chapter Nine: Modified Prescriptions for the Universal Treatment of Fall & Strike Injuries 125

199. Rx for Static Blood Congealed in the Chest Due to Injury
200. Rx for the Treatment of Injury of the Heart Attacked by the Blood with Qi on the Verge of Exhaustion
201. Rx ... Injury within the Heart Attacked by the Qi
202. Rx ... Qi Panting (*i.e.*, Asthma) Due to Injury
203. Rx ... Raving Caused by Martial Injury
204. Rx ... Loss of Hearing Due to Injury
205. Rx ... Qi Obstruction Due to Injury
206. Rx ... Fever Due to Injury
207. Rx ... Blood Stasis Due to Injury
208. Rx ... Mania Due to Injury
209. Rx ... Low Back Pain Due to Martial Injury
210. Rx ... Stools Not Free-flowing (*i.e.*, Constipation) Due to Injury
211. Rx ... Urine Not Free-flowing Due to Injury
212. Rx ... Hemafecia Due to Injury
213. Rx ... Hematuria Due to Injury
214. Rx ... Stools & Urine Not Free-flowing Due to Injury
215. Rx ... Urinary Incontinence Due to Injury
216. Rx ... Fecal Incontinence Due to Injury
217. Rx ... Chilly Pain in the Intestines Due to Injury

218. Rx ... Cough Due to Injury
219. Rx ... Pain in the Right Lower Abdomen Due to Injury
220. Rx ... Hematemesis Due to Injury
221. Rx ... Bad Smell Emanating from the Mouth Due to Injury
222. Rx ... Hearing Not Clear Due to Shortening of the Tongue Due to Detriment & Damage
223. Rx ... Elongated Tongue Due to Injury
224. Rx ... Hiccough Due to Injury
225. Rx ... Bleeding from the 9 Portals Due to Injury
226. Rx ... Difficulty in Turning Body to the Side Due to Injury
227. Rx ... Loss of Consciousness Due to Injury
228. Rx ... Heart Attacked by Qi & Blood Due to Injury
229. Rx ... Splitting Headache Due to Injury
230. Rx ... Headache at the Vertex Due to Injury
231. Rx ... Redness & Swelling of the Eyes Due to Injury
232. Rx ... Nosebleed Due to Broken Nose Due to Martial Injury
233. Rx ... Bleeding from the Ears Due to Martial Injury
234. Rx ... Injury to the Throat Due to Fighting
235. Rx ... Cheek Injury Due to Fighting
236. Rx ... Split Lips Due to Fighting
237. Rx ... Loss of Teeth Due to Fighting
238. Rx ... Loose Teeth Due to Fighting
239. Rx ... Shoulder Pain Due to Fighting
240. Rx ... Pain of the Arm & Hand Due to Fighting
241. Rx ... Injury of the Chest Due to Fighting
242. Rx ... Injury of the Left Ribs Due to Fighting
243. Rx ... Injury of the Right Ribs Due to Fighting
244. Rx ... Abdominal Injury Due to Fighting
245. Rx ... Injury of the Upper Back Due to Fighting
246. Rx ... Low Back Injury Due to   Fighting
247. Rx ... Shooting Pain from the Lower to Upper Back Due to Fighting
248. Rx ... Bilateral Hip Pain Due to Fighting
249. Rx ... Injury of Kidneys Due to Fighting
250. Rx ... Anal Bleeding Due to Fighting
251. Rx ... Swelling & Pain of the Leg Due to Fighting
252. Rx ... Heel Injury Due to Fighting
253. Rx ... Joint Injury Due to Fighting
254. Rx ... Swelling & Pain Due to Static Blood, Accumulations & Gatherings Due to Fighting
255. Rx ... fever & poor appetite Due to Fighting
256. Rx ... Persistent Local Swelling Due to Fighting

257. Rx ... Local Bruise, Swelling & Aversion to Cold Due to Fighting
258. Rx ... Sallow Complexion, Persistent Greenish Swelling, & Alternating Fever & Chills Due to Fighting
259. Rx ... Paraplegia
260. Rx ... Absence of Facial Lustre Due to Fighting

Chapter Ten: Shaolin Training Herbal Prescriptions 139

261. Quiet the Spirit & Tranquilize the Brain Formula
262. Harmonize & Regulate the Qi Mechanism Formula
263. Shaolin Training Formula
264. Soothing the Sinews Elixir
265. Training Wine
266. Unimpeded, Free-flowing Qi & Blood Training Powder
267. Shaolin Good Luck Elixir
268. Harvest the Training Powder

Appendix 145

Index 147

Chapter One

Emergency Formulas For Martial Injuries

1. Shao Lin Fu Mai San
Shao Lin Recover the Pulse Powder

Ingredients: Secretio Moschi Moschiferi (*She Xiang*) 0.3g, Eupolyphaga Seu Opisthoplatia (*Tu Bie Chong*), 7.5g, defatted Semen Crotonis Tiglii (*Ba Dou Shuang*), 3g, Styrax (*Su He Xiang*), 0.9g, Pyritum (*Zi Ran Tong*, dipped in vinegar 7 times[1]), 24g, Gummum Olibani (*Ru Xiang*, vinegar processed[2]), 3g, Myrrha (*Mo Yao*, vinegar processed), 3g, Cinnabar (*Zhu Sha*), 3g, Radix Saussureae Seu Vladimiriae (*Mu Xiang*), 3g, Sanguis Draconis (*Xue Jie*), 3g

Method of preparation: Grind the above 10 ingredients into a fine powder. Mix well and store in a tightly sealed bottle for use.

Method of administration: For an adult, take 0.6-1.2g per time. If

---

[1] Moisten the powdered Pyritum with vinegar and allow to sit in the open air. A green rust will form. Do this seven times, thereby dissolving a certain amount of the copper so that it can enter solution.

[2] For processing 50 kilograms Frankincense, use 2.5 kilograms of vinegar. Crush the Frankincense, fry, and while frying, sprinkle with vinegar. Dry the Frankincense and then recrush it for use.

taken with yellow wine (*i.e.*, rice wine), the results will be better. This prescription can also be used externally for the treatment of wounds by mixing the powder with fresh roasted sesame oil, forming a paste. Such a paste applied to the affected area will bring about an ideal result.

Functions: Arouses the spirit, opens the portals, frees the flow of yang, and restores the pulse.

It is indicated for spirit dimness (*i.e.*, blurring of consciousness), qi inversion, sudden fainting, and loss of consciousness of human affairs. When used externally, it is indicated for all kinds of injury due to fall and strike resulting in localized redness, swelling, aching, and pain.

2. *Shao Lin Xing Jun San*
Shaolin Troop Deployment Powder

Ingredients: Menthol (*Bo He Bing*), 0.3g, persimmon frost (*Shi Shuang*), 1g, Fructus Citri Seu Ponciri (*Zhi Qiao*), 30g, Herba Agastaches Seu Pogostemi (*Huo Xiang*), 30g, Pericarpium Citri Reticulatae (*Chen Pi*), 15g, processed Rhizoma Pinelliae Ternatae (*Ban Xia*), 9g, Radix Achyranthis Bidentatae (*Niu Xi*), 9g, Guangdong Radix Saussureae Seu Vladimiriae (*Guang Mu Xiang*), 9g, Massa Medica Fermentata (*Shen Qu*), 30g, dry Rhizoma Zingiberis (*Gan Jiang*), 6g, Radix Platycodi Grandiflori (*Jie Geng*), 30g, Semen Sterculiae Scaphigeriae (*Pang Da Hai*), 30g, Benzoin (*An Xi Xiang*) 1g, Secretio Moschi Moschiferi (*She Xiang*), 1g, Fructus Crataegi (*Shan Zha*), 30g, raw Radix Glycyrrhizae Uralensis (*Sheng Gan Cao*) 9g.

Method of preparation: Grind the above 16 ingredients into a fine powder according to traditional Chinese procedure. Mix them together until well blended and store in an air-tight, porcelain container. Store until needed in a cool dry place.

Method of administration: For an adult, take 0.3-0.45g (of powder) mixed with either yellow wine (*i.e.*, rice wine) or cold, boiled water.

Functions: Clears heat and relieves summerheat, engenders fluids and stops thirst, fortifies the stomach, and disperses food, dispels phlegm and arouses the spirit. It is mainly used for the treatment of sudden syncope due to summerheat stroke manifesting as lack of consciousness of human affairs, dry mouth and parched tongue, swelling and pain of the throat, no desire for food or drink, nausea, vomiting, chest oppression, hiccup, lockjaw, oral sores, etc.

Commentary: According to the story told by Zhen Jun, teacher of the Patriarch De Chan, this is one of the best commonly used prescriptions for the monk troops in their fighting and marching and has been used for generations. According to the original secret manuscript, during the *Jia Jing* period of the Ming Dynasty, the emperor issued an order to the Shaolin Monastery to set out on an expedition due to frequent invasions along the Chinese southeast coast by Japanese troops. A group of monk soldiers led by Monk Yue Kong was sent out. Because most of the monks were northerners, they were unaccustomed to the climate after marching a thousand *li* into the hot south. Most of the monk soldiers took sick, some of them even critically. It was at this point that the Chief Monk Yue Kong created this prescription. Since it proved so effective in treating those sick monk soldiers, it has ever since been called Shaolin Troop Deployment Powder.

3. Shao Lin Zhen Yu San
Shaolin Precious Jade Powder

Ingredients: Rhizoma Gastrodiae Elatae (*Ming Tian Ma*), Radix Et Rhizoma Notopterygii (*Qiang Huo*), Radix Ledebouriellae Sesloidis (*Fang Feng*), Rhizoma Arisaematis (*Nan Xing*, stir-fried in ginger juice), Radix Angelicae Dahuricae (*Bai Zhi*) 15g each, Rhizoma

Typhonii Gigantei Seu Radix Aconiti Coreani (*Bai Fu Zi*), 3g.

Method of preparation: Grind the above 6 ingredients into a fine powder. Place the resulting powder into a porcelain jar and seal as tightly as possible.

Method of administration: Take 0.2-0.3g of powder each time mixed with yellow wine (*i.e.*, rice wine) or cold, boiled water.

Functions: Arouses the spirit and frees the flow of yang, opens the portals and settles tetany. It is indicated for lack of consciousness of human affairs, deviation of the mouth and eyes, and convulsions due to all kinds of fall and strike, detriment and injury. Externally, it is applicable to ulcerated wounds.

Commentary: According to the manuscript, this prescription possesses the effect of revitalization. If a slight warmth can still be felt in the patient's precordial region, the patient can be brought back to life after taking 9g of this powder. However, if there is vomiting, which is not usual, a cure (by this prescription) will be more difficult.

4. First Aid Prescription for Hematemesis Due to Injury to the Precordium

Ingredients: Rhizoma Bletillae Striatae (*Bai Ji*), 30g, Radix Pseudoginseng (*San Qi*), 0.6g, Crinis Carbonisatus (*Xue Yu Tan*), 9g, carbonized Fructus Gardeniae Jasminoidis (*Zhi Zi Tan*), 15g, carbonized Radix Et Rhizoma Rhei (*Da Huang Tan*), 9g, stir-fried Radix Albus Paeoniae Lactiflorae (*Bai Shao*), Herba Verbenae (*Ma Deng Cao*), 30g.

Method of administration: Grind the above medicinals into a fine powder. Take 9g internally.

Note: *Ma Deng Cao* is a grass grown on Song Shan which is known for its specific hemostatic effect.

5. Prescription for the Treatment of Fainting Due to Injury to *Bai Hui* (GV 20)

Ingredients: Radix Praeparatus Aconiti Carmichaeli (*Fu Zi*), 9g, Rhizoma Atractylodis Macrocephalae (*Bai Zhu*), 12g, mix-fried Radix Astragali Membranacei (*Huang Qi*), 30g, Rhizoma Acori Graminei (*Chang Pu*), 9g, Styrax (*Su He Xiang*), 0.9g, dry Rhizoma Zingiberis (*Gan Jiang*), 3 slices

Method of administration: Decoct to get 1 soupbowlful (of medicinal liquid). Take internally for an instantaneous result.

6. *Shao Lin Duo Ming San*
Shaolin Seizing Life Powder

Ingredients: Processed Radix Aconiti Chinensis (*Cao Wu*), Gummum Olibani (*Ru Xiang*, vinegar processed), Myrrha (*Mo Yao*, vinegar processed), Sanguis Draconis (*Xue Jie*), & Pyritum (*Zi Ran Tong*, dipped 7 times in vinegar), each in equal portions

Method of preparation: Grind the above 5 medicinals into a fine powder and store them in a bottle until use.

Method of administration: Take 6g each time with yellow wine (*i.e.*, rice wine).

7. *Er Wei Fu Sheng San*
Two Flavors Recover Life Powder

Ingredients: Raw Rhizoma Pinelliae Ternatae (*Sheng Ban Xia*), raw Radix Et Rhizoma Rhei (*Sheng Da Huang*), each in equal portions

Method of preparation: Grind the above ingredients into a fine powder for use.

Method of use: Blow the appropriate amount of powder into the patient's nose, the left nostril for a male and the right nostril for a female.

Functions: Opens the portals and arouses the spirit. It is mainly used for qi inversion, fright inversion, and lack of consciousness of human affairs due to fall and strike, detriment and injury.

Commentary: Nasal pain will be felt when the patient regains consciousness. Application of ginger juice will relieve this pain after some time.

8. Treatment for Unstoppable Hematemesis

Ingredients: Radix Angelicae Sinensis (*Dang Gui*), 18g, raw Radix Albus Paeoniae Lactiflorae (*Sheng Bai Shao*), 9g, Gelatinum Corii Asini (*E Jiao*), 12g, Rhizoma Bletillae Striatae (*Bai Ji*), 9g, Flos Carthami Tinctorii (*Hong Hua*), 3g, Radix Platycodi Grandiflori (*Jie Geng*), 8g, stir-fried Fructus Citri Seu Ponciri (*Zhi Qiao*), 6g, Radix Pseudoginseng (*Tian San Qi*), 3g, Radix Rehmanniae (*Sheng Di*), 30g, blackened Herba Seu Flos Schizonepetae Tenuifoliae (*Hei Jing Jie*), 12g, Pulvis Fumi Carbonisati (*Bai Cao Shuang*), 9g, red sugar (*i.e.*, brown sugar, *Hong Tang*), 30g

Decoct in water and take. Typically, 2 *ji* will cure (the patient).

Commentary: Fairly good results can be achieved (with this formula) in the treatment of all kinds of hemorrhagic conditions due to external injury.

9. Fu Mai Tang
Recover the Pulse Decoction

Ingredients: Radix Panacis Ginseng (*Ren Shen*), 30g, mix-fried Radix Astragali Membranacei (*Huang Qi*), 9g, Rhizoma Atractylodis Macrocephalae (*Bai Zhu*), 9g, Radix Praeparatus Aconiti Carmichaeli (*Fu Zi*), 3g

Method of administration: Decoct in water and take. Fairly good effect.

Functions: Supplements the qi, returns the yang, and restores the pulse

10. Wu Bao Dan
Five Treasure Elixir

Ingredients: Calculus Bovis (*Niu Huang*), 3g, Secretio Moschi Moschiferi (*She Xiang*), 0.6g, Succinum (*Hu Po*), 6g, Pulvis Cornu Rhinocerotis (*Xi Jiao Fen*), 6g, Benzoin (*An Xi Xiang*), 9g

Method of preparation: Grind the above 5 medicinal ingredients into an extremely fine powder. Make pills the size of mung beans after the powder is mixed with mung bean powder. Store the pills in a bottle for use.

Method of administration: For adults, take 3g internally each time with ginger soup (*Jiang Tang*) for a good effect.

Functions: Clears heat and resolves toxins, opens the portals and arouses the brain

This formula produces fairly good results in the treatment of critical conditions, such as coma and qi inversion due to summerheat stroke, paralysis, and all kinds of detriment and injury.

Commentary: This is a secret empirical prescription created by Patriarch De Chan on the basis of his scores of years of experience. It can be used not only in the treatment of the above mentioned conditions, but also in cases of acute and chronic infantile convulsions and fetid vomiting.

Chapter Two

Stop Bleeding Formulas

11. *Shao Lin Zhi Xue San*
Shaolin Stop Bleeding Powder

Ingredients: Radix Pseudoginseng (*San Qi*), 9g, Crinis Carbonisatus (*Xue Yu Tan*), 9g, Rhizoma Bletillae Striatae (*Bai Ji*), 15g, Herba Verbenae (*Ma Deng Cao*), 24g

Grind the above 4 ingredients into a fine powder. Add a small amount of Borneol (*Bing Pian*) and keep in a bottle for use. For bleeding due to external injury, sprinkle some of this powder over the wound and it will immediately stop the bleeding.

12. *San Bao Zhi Xue San*
Three Treasures Stop Bleeding Powder

Ingredients: Fructificatio Lasiospherae (*Ma Bo*), 30g, Cortex Phellodendri (*Huang Bai*), 30g, Radix Pseudoginseng (*San Qi*), 9g

Grind the above 3 herbs into a fine powder. In case of local bleeding due to knife wound, apply this powder to the affected area.

13. Shao Lin Jin Shang San
Shaolin Metal Injury Powder

Ingredients: Myrrha (*Mo Yao*), 15g, Gummum Olibani (*Ru Xiang*), 15g, Sanguis Draconis (*Xue Jie*), 9g, Lignum Sappanis (*Su Mu*), 9g, Radix Angelicae Sinensis (*Dang Gui*), 24g, Os Draconis (*Long Gu*), 15g, powdered Radix Pseudoginseng (*San Qi Fen*), 30g

Method of preparation: Place the first 6 ingredients in a porcelain jar and cover with a lid. Seal the lid with mud. Then bake in a mild fire for 45 minutes. After the temperature has cooled, remove the ingredients and grind them into powder. Mix this powder with the Pseudoginseng powder and store in a bottle for use.

Method of use: Reliable results can be achieved in case of bleeding due to external injury when this powder is applied to the affected area.

14. Yang Family Spear Wound Powder

Ingredients: Secretio Moschi Moschiferi (*She Xiang*), 1.5g, Acacia Catechu (*Er Cha*), 60g, Myrrha (*Mo Yao*, vinegar processed), 30g, Gummum Olibani (*Ru Xiang*, vinegar processed), 30g, Cinnabar (*Zhu Sha*, ground with water[1]), 30g, Herba Verbenae *Ma Deng Cao*), 30g, Rhizoma Bletillae Striatae (*Bai Ji*), 30g, Sanguis Draconis (*Xue Jie*), 24g, Semen Pruni Persicae (*Tao Ren*), 30g, Radix Rubrus Paeoniae Lactiflorae (*Chi Shao*), 30g, raw Radix Glycyrrhizae (*Sheng Gan Cao*), 15g.

Method of preparation: Grind the above 11 ingredients (except the Musk) into a fine powder. Divide into packets each containing 1.5g

---

[1] Grinding Cinnabar under water reduces this ingredient's toxicity.

Stop Bleeding Formulas

of powder and store these in an air-tight container.

Method of use: For adults, 1 packet should be taken each time with yellow wine (*i.e.*, rice wine). Externally, the powder can be applied to the affected area to staunch bleeding from a knife wound. In case of an ulcerated wound, mix the powder with fresh roasted sesame oil (*Sheng Xiang You*) into a paste and apply the paste to the affected area. Such a wound will be cured in from 2-3 days.

Functions: Disperses swelling, stops pain, stops bleeding, stops itching, and resolves toxins. This formula is indicated for local hemorrhage, redness, swelling, pain, and ulceration due to wounds caused by iron weapons, such as broadswords and spearheads.

15. Rx for the Treatment of Bleeding Due to Injury of the Nose

Quickly smash several fresh Folium Perillae Frutescentis (*Zi Su Ye*) and pack the nostrils with this. The bleeding will be checked instantly.

16. Rx for the Treatment of Nose Bleed

Grind some Crinis Carbonisatus (*Xue Yu Tan*) into a fine powder and put in the nose. At the same time, apply a cold water compress to the forehead.

17. Rx for the Treatment of Hematuria Due to Injury of the Lower Abdomen

Ingredients: Carbonized Herba Cephalanoplos Segeti (*Xiao Ji*), 30g, Rhizoma Imperatae Cylindricae (*Bai Mao Gen*), 30g, Radix Pseudoginseng (*San Qi*), 0.9g, Herba Dianthi (*Qu Mai*), 30g, Semen

Malvae Verticillatae (*Dong Kui Zi*), 15g, Crinis Carbonisatus (*Xue Yu Tan*), 15g

Method of administration: Decoct the above 7 medicinal ingredients down into 1 bowlful. Add to this 1 cup of infant's urine. Take the powdered Pseudoginseng separately (*i.e.*, do not decoct with the other ingredients).[2]

18. Rx for the Treatment of Hemafecia Due to Injury of the Lower Abdomen

Ingredients: Raw Radix Sanguisorbae (*Sheng Di Yu*), 30g, Radix Rehmanniae (*Sheng Di*), 30g, Sichuan Rhizoma Coptidis Chinensis (*Chuan Huang Lian*), 9g, Radix Puerariae Lobatae (*Ge Gen*), 30g, 1 handful of Fructus Forsythiae Suspensae (*Lian Qiao*), carbonized Flos Immaturus Sophorae Japonicae (*Huai Hua Tan*), 15g, raw Radix Glycyrrhizae (*Sheng Gan Cao*), 6g

Decoct with water. Results will be seen after taking 2 *ji*.

19. Rx for Treatment of Bleeding from the 7 Portals Due to Injury[3]

Ingredients: Carbonized Radix Angelicae Sinensis (*Dang Gui Tan*), Crinis Carbonisatus (*Xue Yu Tan*), carbonized Fructus Gardeniae Jasminoidis (*Zhi Zi Tan*), carbonized Cortex Phellodendri (*Huang Bai Tan*), carbonized Radix Et Rhizoma Rhei (*Da Huang Tan*), 9g each,

---

[2] Raw Pseudoginseng has a different property than if it is cooked. Raw, it relieves stagnation and is a hemostatic. Cooked, it is a blood tonic.

[33] *I.e.*, eyes, ears, both nostrils, and mouth

Radix Rehmanniae (*Sheng Di*), 30g, Radix Pseudoginseng (*San Qi*), 1.5g (take separately).

Decoct in water and take.

20. Rx for the Treatment of Bleeding from the Eye

Ingredients: Carbonized Pollen Typhae (*Pu Huang Tan*), 9g, Rhizomatis Nelumbinis Nuciferae (*Ou Jie*), 30g, Rhizoma Imperatae Cylindricae (*Bai Mao Gen*), 30g, Radix Rehmanniae (*Sheng Di*), 30g, Folium Lopthatheri Gracilis (*Da Zhu Ye*), 9g, Herba Equiseti Hiemalis (*Mu Zei*), 12g, Fructus Tribuli Terrestris (*Bai Ji Li*), 30g, Sichuan Rhizoma Coptidis Chinensis (*Chuan Huang Lian*), 6g, Flos Chrysanthemi Morifolii (*Ju Hua*), 6g

Decoct in water and take. Two to 3 *ji* will cure.

21. Shao Lin Wan Nang Zhi Xue San
Shaolin Ten Thousand Abilities Stop Bleeding Powder

Ingredients: Fructificatio Lasiosphaerae (*Ma Bo*), 30g, Radix Rehmanniae (*Sheng Di*), 30g, Rhizoma Bletillae Striatae (*Bai Ji*), 30g, Flos Lonicerae Japonicae (*Jin Yin Hua*), 30g, Crinis Carbonisatus (*Xue Yu Tan*), 15g, raw Radix Et Rhizoma Rhei (*Sheng Da Huang*), raw Fructus Gardeniae Jasminoidis (*Sheng Zhi Zi*), raw Cortex Phellodendri (*Sheng Huang Bai*), raw Rhizoma Coptidis Chinensis (*Sheng Huang Lian*), 9g each, Acacia Catechu (*Er Cha*), 15g, Gummum Olibani (*Ru Xiang*, vinegar processed), Myrrha (*Mo Yao*, vinegar processed), 12g each, Sanguis Draconis (*Xue Jie*), 10g, Pyritum (*Zi Ran Tong*, dipped in vinegar 7 times), 15g, Secretio Moschi Moschiferi (*She Xiang*), 3g, Borneol (*Bing Pian*), 3g

Method of preparation: Grind the above 16 medicinals into a fine powder and keep them in a bottle for use.

Method of use: Application of this powder to a bleeding wound due to local injury is capable of stopping pain and stopping bleeding. In case of internal injury and blood stasis, take 6-9g of powder internally with either yellow wine (*i.e.*, rice wine) or infant's urine. If the affected area is ulcerous and recalcitrant to heal, a paste made from fresh roasted sesame oil (*Sheng Xiang You*) should be applied to the ulcer and some of the powder should also be taken internally at the same time for better effect.

Functions: Clears heat and resolves toxins, disperses swelling and stops pain, stops bleeding and transforms stasis, dispels pus and engenders (new) tissue

Indications: Hemorrhage due to internal and external injury, pain, and ulcerous skin toxins

Chapter Three

Fall, Strike, Bruise & Contusion Formulas

22. Rx for the Treatment of Bruises & Swelling Due to External Injury

Ingredients: Flos Carthami Tinctorii (*Hong Hua*), 6g, Radix Rubrus Paeoniae Lactiflorae (*Chi Shao*), 15g, Semen Pruni Persicae (*Tao Ren*), 3g, Pyritum (*Zi Ran Tong*, dipped in vinegar 7 times), 0.9g, Radix Angelicae Sinensis (*Dang Gui*), 15g, Radix Saussureae Seu Vladimiriae (*Mu Xiang*), 3g, raw Radix Glycyrrhizae (*Sheng Gan Cao*), 3g

Decoct in water, mix with yellow wine (*i.e.*, rice wine), and take. A good result can be expected.

23. Rx for the Treatment of Insidious Pain of the Chest & Lateral Costal Area Caused by Hit by Fist

Ingredients: Semen Pruni Persicae (*Tao Ren*), 6g, Flos Carthami Tinctorii (*Hong Hua*), 9g, Tuber Curcumae (*Yu Jin*), 3g, Yunnan Radix Saussureae Seu Vladimiriae (*Yun Mu Xiang*), 4.5g, Lignum Sappanis (*Su Mu*), 9g, Eupolyphaga Seu Opisthoplatia (*Tu Bie Chong*), 3g, Pyritum (*Zi Ran Tong*, dipped in vinegar 7 times), 1.5g, Radix Angelicae Sinensis (*Dang Gui*), 15g, Rhizoma Ligustici

Wallichii (*Chuan Xiong*), 9g, Radix Rubrus Paeoniae Lactiflorae (*Chi Shao*), 9g, Radix Albus Paeoniae Lactiflorae (*Bai Shao*), 9g

Method of administration: Decoct the above 11 medicinals in 3000ml of cold spring water (*Qing Quan Shui*) until reduced to 500ml. Mix the resulting juice with 1 cup infant's urine (male, firstborn).

24. Rx for the Treatment of Pain of the Lower Abdomen Due to Hit

Ingredients: Radix Angelicae Sinensis (*Dang Gui*), 15g, Rhizoma Ligustici Wallichii (*Chuan Xiong*), 6g, Rhizoma Cyperi Rotundi (*Xiang Fu*), 9g, Rhizoma Corydalis Yanhusuo (*Yan Hu Suo*), 9g, Radix Saussureae Seu Vladimiriae (*Mu Xiang*), 4.5g, Radix Rubrus Paeoniae Lactiflorae (*Chi Shao*), 9g, Semen Pruni Persicae (*Tao Ren*), 6g, Radix Salviae Miltiorrhizae (*Dan Shen*), 30g, Feces Trogopterori Seu Pteromi (*Wu Ling Zhi*), 6g, raw Pollen Typhae (*Sheng Pu Huang*), 4.5g

Decoct the above medicinals in water and take.

25. Rx for the Treatment of Injury to the Sinews Due to Fist or Weapon

Ingredients: Freshwater crab (*Pang Xie*), 1 piece, several pieces old (*i.e.*, large) snails (*Lao Wo Niu*)

Smash both into a paste and apply to the affected area. Bandage with white gauze.

26. Technique for the Treatment of Dislocation of the Jaw

The patient should be instructed to sit in a chair. One monk should hold the jaw with both hands. Then push with force in the natural direction until it enters its natural position. Then smash Rhizoma Arisaematis (*Nan Xing*) and spread on a white cloth. Apply this cloth to the affected area (*i.e.*, the temporomandibular joint).

27. Rx for the Treatment of Swelling & Pain of the Face Due to Hit Injury

Ingredients: Semen Momordicae Cochinensis (*Mu Bie Zi*) 3 pieces (should be burned into an ash & mixed with roasted sesame oil [*Xiang You*]), some Pyrolusite (*Wu Ming Yi*), Pyritum (*Zi Ran Tong*, dipped in vinegar 7 times), 3g, Gummum Olibani (*Ru Xiang*, remove the oil), 9g, Myrrha (*Mo Yao*, remove the oil), 9g, Lignum Sappanis (*Su Mu*), 9g

Method of preparation: Grind the above medicinals into a fine powder. Make into pills the size of a marble with honey and take 3 pills each time, washed down with white alcohol (*i.e.*, clear alcohol).

Note: Pyrolusite is a type of black sand grain found in yellow earth.

28. Rx for the Treatment of Localized Incessant Pain Due to Hit Injury

Ingredients: Rhizoma Gastrodiae Elatae (*Tian Ma*), 9g, Radix Angelicae Dahuricae (*Bai Zhi*), 9g, Rhizoma Typhonii Gigantei Seu Radix Aconiti Coreani (*Bai Fu Zi*), 9g, raw Rhizoma Arisaematis (*Sheng Nan Xing*), 9g, Radix Ledebouriellae Sesloidis (*Fang Feng*), 9g

Method of preparation: Grind the above medicinals into powder, add *Shi Xiao San* (Loss of Smile Powder)[1], 30g, and mix together.

Method of administration: Take 9g each time together with 30g of yellow wine (*i.e.*, rice wine). If this powdered medicine is also used externally after mixing with vinegar, the effect will be better.

29. Rx for the Treatment of Injury to the Sinews Due to Fist & Stick

Two snails (*Wo Niu*), one crab's carapace (*Xie Tou*), fresh Herba Cum Radice Taraxaci Mongolici (*Xian Gong Ying*), 30g

Smash into a paste, add a little Borneol (*Bing Pian*), and apply to the affected area. One will recover in 3 days.

30. Rx for the Treatment of Bruise & Swelling Due to Injury by Fist

Fat pork (*Pang Zhu Rou*), 250g, day lily buds (*Huang Hua Cai*), 500g[2]

Smash into a paste, add a small amount of Borneol (*Bing Pian*), and apply to the affected area.

---

[1] *I.e.*, Feces Trogopterori Seu Pteromi (*Wu Ling Zhi*) 10-15g and Pollen Typhae (*Pu Huang*) 10-15g

[2] If using dry day lily buds, called Golden Needles colloquially, they should be reconstituted by soaking in water before smashing.

31. Rx for the Treatment of Insidious Pain of the Precordium Due to Strike by Fist

Ingredients: Tabanus (*Meng Chong*, remove the wings), 5 bugs, Cortex Radicis Moutan (*Dan Pi*), 30g, Flos Carthami Tinctorii (*Hong Hua*), 15g, Radix Albus Paeoniae Lactiflorae (*Bai Shao*), 15g

Decoct in water and add 1 cup of infant's urine. Take internally.

32. Rx for the Treatment of Injury to the Head

Ingredients: Radix Rehmanniae (*Sheng Di*), 45g, Radix Panacis Ginseng (*Ren Shen*), 6g, Camphora (*Long Nao*), 1.2g, Dens Draconis (*Long Chi*), 15g, Cortex Elephantis (*Xiang Pi*), 15g, Radix Astragali Membranacei (*Huang Qi*), 30g

Grind into powder. Take 3g each time, 3 times per day.

33. Rx for the Treatment of Chest Pain Due to Fist Injury

Ingredients: Rhizoma Corydalis Yanhusuo (*Yan Hu Suo*), 6g, Flos Carthami Tinctorii (*Hong Hua*), 15g, Cortex Populi Suaveolentis (*Qing Yang Shu Pi*), 60g, Ramulus Pruni Persicae (*Tao Zhi*), 30g

Decoct in water and take. If infant's urine is added, the effect will be better.

34. Rx for the Treatment of Headache at the Corner of the Forehead Due to Fist Hit

Ingredients: Radix Angelicae Sinensis (*Dang Gui*), 30g, Rhizoma Ligustici Wallichii (*Chuan Xiong*), 9g, Radix Albus Paeoniae Lactiflorae (*Bai Shao*), 9g, wild goat horn (*Shan Yang Jiao*, powder & take separately), 9g, Herba Cum Radice Asari (*Xi Xin*), 3g, Flos

Carthami Tinctorii (*Hong Hua*), 15g, Semen Pruni Persicae (*Tao Ren*), 9g, Radix Glycyrrhizae (*Gan Cao*) 3g

Decoct in water and take.

35. Rx for the Treatment of Insidious Pain of the Lower Abdomen Due to Fist Hit

Ingredients: Radix Angelicae Sinensis (*Dang Gui*), 15g, Flos Carthami Tinctorii (*Hong Hua*), 9g, Tabanus (*Meng Chong*, remove the wings & legs), 1.5g, raw Pollen Typhae (*Sheng Pu Huang*), 6g, Feces Trogopterori Seu Pteromi (*Wu Ling Zhi*, vinegar processed), 6g

Decoct in water and take.

36. Rx for the Treatment of Low Back Pain Due to Injury by Stick

Ingredients: Radix Angelicae Sinensis (*Dang Gui*), 30g, Flos Carthami Tinctorii (*Hong Hua*), 9g, Rhizoma Ligustici Wallichii (*Chuan Xiong*), 9g, Pyritum (*Zi Ran Tong*, dipped in vinegar 7 times) 6g, Radix Cyathulae (*Chuan Niu Xi*), 15g, Caulis Millettiae Seu Spatholobi (*Ji Xue Teng*), 30g, Lignum Sappanis (*Su Mu*), 9g, Radix Et Rhizoma Rhei (*Da Huang*), 9g

Decoct in water and take.

37. Rx for the Treatment of Swelling & Pain of the Nape of the Neck Due to Injury by Stick

Ingredients: Semen Pruni Armeniacae (*Xing Ren*), 5 kernels, Semen Pruni Persicae (*Tao Ren*), 10 kernels, Sichuan Rhizoma Coptidis Chinensis (*Chuan Huang Lian*), 15g, Sanguis Draconis (*Xue Jie*), 1.5g, Fructus Zanthoxyli Bungeani (*Chuan Jiao*), 0.9g

Fall, Strike, Bruise & Contusion Formulas

Smash the above ingredients into a paste and apply to the affected area.

38. Rx for the Treatment of Headache of the Forehead Due to Hit by Stick

Ingredients: Radix Angelicae Dahuricae (*Bai Zhi*), Radix Pseudoginseng (*San Qi*), Alum (*Bai Fan*), Galla Rhi Chinensis (*Wu Bei Zi*), each in equal amounts

Grind into powder and mix with raw sesame oil (*Sheng Xiang You*) into a paste. Apply to the affected area. It will stop the pain instantaneously.

39. Rx for the Treatment of Swelling & Pain of the Shoulder Due to Hit of Whip

Ingredients: Radix Angelicae Sinensis (*Dang Gui*), 15g, Rhizoma Ligustici Wallichii (*Chuan Xiong*), 9g, raw Pollen Typhae (*Sheng Pu Huang*), 3g, Fructus Zanthoxyli Bungeani (*Chuan Jiao*), 0.6g, Herba Lycopi Lucidi (*Ze Lan*), 9g, Flos Carthami Tinctorii (*Hong Hua*), 9g, Semen Pruni Persicae (*Tao Ren*), 9g

Decoct in water and then add 1 cup of infant's urine. Take internally.

40. Rx for the Treatment of Injury of Body Due to Hit of Stick & Sudden Fall

Ingredients: Gelatinum Corii Asini (*Lu Pi Gao*), 30g, aged Folium Artimisiae Argyii (*Chen Ai Ye*), 6g, Flos Carthami Tinctorii (*Hong Hua*), 9g, Radix Rubrus Paeoniae Lactiflorae (*Chi Shao*), 9g

Decoct in water. Yellow wine (*i.e.*, rice wine) can be added to guide the properties of the other ingredients. In that case, the effect of the whole formula will be better.

41. Rx for the Treatment of Pain in the Right Lateral Costal Area Due to Fist Strike

Ingredients: Gummum Olibani (*Ru Xiang*, vinegar processed), Myrrha (*Mo Yao*, vinegar processed), 4.5g each, Radix Angelicae Sinensis (*Dang Gui*), 15g, Pyritum (*Zi Ran Tong*, dipped in vinegar 7 times), 1.5g, Flos Carthami Tinctorii (*Hong Hua*), Radix Rubrus Paeoniae Lactiflorae (*Chi Shao*), Lignum Sappanis (*Su Mu*), 9g each, Tuber Curcumae (*Yu Jin*), 6g, Sanguis Draconis (*Xue Jie*), 1.5g, Radix Glycyrrhizae (*Gan Cao*), 4.5g

Decoct in 2000ml of water and reduce to 500ml. Add 1 cup of infant's urine and take internally.

42. Rx for the Treatment of Pain of the Right Lateral Costal Area

Ingredients: Gummum Olibani (*Ru Xiang*, vinegar processed), Myrrha (*Mo Yao*, vinegar processed), 9g each, Camphora (*Long Nao*), 1.2g, Sanguis Draconis (*Xue Jie*), 6g, raw Radix Glycyrrhizae (*Sheng Gan Cao*), 3g, Borneol (*Bing Pian*), 3g, Alum (*Bai Fan*), 6g

Grind the above medicinals into a fine powder. If the skin is ruptured, apply these ingredients to the affected area. This is effective for stopping pain and bleeding. If the skin is not broken but is only red, swollen, and painful, mix the above ingredients with roasted sesame oil (*Xiang You*) and apply to the affected area. The patient will be cured in 1-2 days.

Fall, Strike, Bruise & Contusion Formulas

43. Rx for the Treatment of Injury Due to Fall Because of Unexpected Push

Ingredients: Radix Angelicae Sinensis (*Dang Gui*), 15g, Rhizoma Ligustici Wallichii (*Chuan Xiong*), 9g, Cortex Cinnamomi (*Rou Gui*), 1.5g, Flos Carthami Tinctorii (*Hong Hua*), 9g, Radix Achyranthis Bidentatae (*Niu Xi*), 15g, Radix Glycyrrhizae (*Gan Cao*), 6g, Gummum Olibani (*Ru Xiang*, vinegar processed), Myrrha (*Mo Yao*, vinegar processed), 4.5g each

Add 1000ml of water and 250ml white alcohol, decoct, and take internally.

44. Jiu Long Tang
Nine Dragon Decoction

Ingredients: Sanguis Draconis (*Xue Jie*), 3g, Acacia Catechu (*Er Cha*), 3g, Flos Carthami Tinctorii (*Hong Hua*), 9g, Radix Angelicae Sinensis (*Dang Gui*), 15g, Radix Rubrus Paeoniae Lactiflorae (*Chi Shao*), 6g, Camphora (*Long Nao*), 0.3g, Cinnabar (*Zhu Sha*), 15g, Cortex Cinnamomi (*Rou Gui*), 1.5g, Radix Praeparatus Aconiti Carmichaeli (*Fu Zi*), 1.5g

Grind the above 9 medicinals into fine powder. Each time take 1g with 30ml of white alcohol. This prescription is indicated for all injuries.

45. Rx for the Treatment of Redness & Swelling Due to Injury by Fist or Stick

Ingredients: Radix Angelicae Sinensis (*Dang Gui*), 15g, Rhizoma Ligustici Wallichii (*Chuan Xiong*), 9g, Flos Carthami Tinctorii (*Hong Hua*), 9g, Pericarpium Citri Reticulati (*Chen Pi*), 6g, Radix Saussureae Seu Vladimiriae (*Mu Xiang*), 4.5g, Fructus Citri Seu

Ponciri (*Zhi Qiao*), 6g, Semen Pruni Persicae (*Tao Ren*), 9g, Caulis Akebiae Mutong (*Mu Tong*), 6g, Gummum Olibani (*Ru Xiang*, vinegar processed), 4.5g, Myrrha (*Mo Yao*, vinegar processed), 4.5g, Radix Glycyrrhizae (*Gan Cao*), 6g

Decoct in water. Then add 30ml of yellow wine (*i.e.*, rice wine) and take. Indicated for all symptoms of internal accumulation of blood stasis.

46. Rx for the Treatment of Skin Rupture in the Area of Injury

Ingredients: Powdered Radix Pseudoginseng (*San Qi Fen*), 9g, Crinis Carbonisatus (*Xue Yu Tan*), 1.5g, Secretio Moschi Moschiferi (*She Xiang*), 0.3g, Radix Angelicae Dahuricae (*Bai Zhi*), 15g, Radix Trichosanthis Kirlowii (*Hua Fen*), 1.5g

Grind the above medicinals into a fine powder and apply to affected area. It will stop bleeding and pain. These ingredients can be taken internally, 1g per time, for the purpose of treating internal hemorrhage.

47. Rx for the Treatment of Ulcerous Lesions in the Area of Injury

Ingredients: Radix Angelicae Sinensis (*Dang Gui*), Rhizoma Ligustici Wallichii (*Chuan Xiong*), Gummum Olibani (*Ru Xiang*, vinegar processed), Myrrha (*Mo Yao*, vinegar processed), 4.5g each, Radix Angelicae Dahuricae (*Bai Zhi*), 9g, Rhizoma Corydalis Yanhusuo (*Yan Hu Suo*), 12g, Radix Glycyrrhizae (*Gan Cao*), 6g, Radix Rubrus Paeoniae Lactiflorae (*Chi Shao*), 9g, Flos Lonicerae Japonicae (*Jin Yin Hua*), 9g, Fructus Forsythiae Suspensae (*Lian Qiao*), 15g, Herba Cum Radice Taraxaci Mongolici (*Pu Gong Ying*), 30g

Decoct in water and take. If 30ml of yellow wine (*i.e.*, rice wine) are added, the effect will be better.

48. Rx for the Treatment of Post Injury Hemorrhagic Dizziness

Ingredients: Radix Panacis Ginseng (*Ren Shen*), 30g, Radix Praeparatus Aconiti Carmichaeli (*Fu Zi*), 9g

Decoct in water and take.

49. Rx for the Treatment of Failure to Generate New (Tissue) in Enduring Ulcerous Wounds

Ingredients: Radix Scutellariae Baicalensis (*Huang Qin*), 6g, Radix Angelicae Dahuricae (*Bai Zhi*), 6g, Radix Trichosanthis Kirlowii (*Tian Hua Fen*), 9g, Calomelas (*Qing Fen*), 0.6g, Gummum Olibani (*Ru Xiang*, vinegar processed), 4.5g, Myrrha (*Mo Yao*, vinegar processed), 4.5g, Flos Lonicerae Japonicae (*Jin Yin Hua*), 4.5g, Fructus Forsythiae Suspensae (*Lian Qiao*), 6g, Secretio Moschi Moschiferi (*She Xiang*), 0.6g, Sanguis Draconis (*Xue Jie*), 9g, Lignum Dalbergiae Odoriferae (*Jiang Xiang*), 6g, Os Draconis (*Long Gu*), 6g, raw Rhizoma Arisaematis (*Sheng Nan Xing*), 6g, nodular iron pyrites (*She Han Shi*), 6g

Grind the above medicinals into a fine powder and mix together well. Keep in a bottle for use. When applied, use just enough to sprinkle over the affected area before bandaging.

Note: Taking internally is strictly prohibited. This powder can be mixed with roasted sesame oil (*Xiang You*) and made into a paste for the treatment of pernicious skin lesions, swelling, and ulceration when applied externally.

50. Rx for the Treatment of Greenish Appearance & Discharge of Pus from Affected Area

Ingredients: Flos Lonicerae Japonicae (*Jin Yin Hua*), 30g, Fructus Forsythiae Suspensae (*Lian Qiao*), 30g, Radix Angelicae Dahuricae (*Bai Zhi*), 9g, Gummum Olibani (*Ru Xiang*, vinegar processed), 6g, Myrrha (*Mo Yao*, vinegar processed), 6g, Radix Astragali Membranacei (*Huang Qi*), 30g, Radix Ledebouriellae Sesloidis (*Fang Feng*), 9g, Radix Rubrus Paeoniae Lactiflorae (*Chi Shao*), 9g, raw Radix Glycyrrhizae (*Sheng Gan Cao*), 6g

Decoct in water.

Commentary: Take all the juice and drink 30ml of highest quality white alcohol. Damp toxins will subside in 2-3 days. The color of the affected area will turn from greenish to red. The patient should take 3-5 *ji* consecutively. During this time, garlic, mutton, and mung bean soup are contraindicated.

51. Rx for the Treatment of Injury to the Head by Stick

Ingredients: Semen Pruni Persicae (*Tao Ren*), 9g, Flos Carthami Tinctorii (*Hong Hua*), 9g, Gummum Olibani (*Ru Xiang*, vinegar processed), 4.5g, Myrrha (*Mo Yao*, vinegar processed), 4.5g, Sanguis Draconis (*Xue Jie*), 4.5g, Radix Angelicae Sinensis (*Dang Gui*), 15g, Eupolyphaga Seu Opisthoplatia (*Tu Bie Chong*), 6g, Pyritum (*Zi Ran Tong*, dipped in vinegar 7 times), 0.9g, Fructus Piperis Albi (*Bai Hu Jiao*, *i.e.*, white peppercorns), 1.8g

Grind the above 8 medicinals into fine powder and then decoct the white pepper in 2000ml spring water until reduced to 1 cup. Then mix the herbal powder with the resulting juice into pills the size of mung beans. Dry and store for use. For adults, take 4.5g each time with yellow wine (*i.e.*, rice wine).

Commentary: According to *Quan Pu (Boxing Manual)*[3], this formula has been secretly passed down by the monks of the Shaolin Monastery. It is effective for all cases of injury to the body by strike of stick. In this case, the skin may be either broken or intact. It is also effective even in extreme cases with qi inversion and unconsciousness. If the skin is broken, the medicinal powder can be sprinkled over the affected area. It will take 3 days for recovery after being bandaged. Use with care during pregnancy.

52. Rx for the Treatment of Neck Hit by Fist

Ingredients: Flos Carthami Tinctorii (*Hong Hua*), 9g, Flos Impatientis Balsaminae (*Feng Xian Hua*), 15g, Flos Chrysanthemi Indici (*Ye Ju Hua*), 30g, Herba Artimisiae Anomalae (*Liu Ji Nu*), 9g, Ramulus Pruni Persicae (*Tao Zhi*), 30g, Ramulus Salicis Babylonicae (*i.e.*, *Liu Shu Zhi*, willow tree twigs), 30g, Ramulus Populi Suaveolentis (*i.e.*, *Qing Yang Shu Zhi*, green poplar tree twigs), 30g, Ramulus Sophorae Japonicae (*Huai Shu Zhi*), 30g

Decoct in water. Two *ji* will produce an effect.

Commentary: Zhen Zu, 29th Patriarch of Shaolin Monastery, once used this formula in the treatment of over 100 patients caused by martial injury. It is also quite effective in the treatment of pernicious skin lesions of the lower extremity. It can be taken internally or used as a fumigant or as a wash.

---

[3] A Shaolin manuscript which is the recording place of many of these formulas

53. Rx for the Treatment of Injury to the Neck Caused by Halberd

In case of instant hemorrhage caused by injury to the neck by halberd, use powdered Radix Pseudoginseng (*San Qi Fen*) and Herba Verbenae (*Ma Deng Cao*) in equal parts and spread over the affected area. This will stop the bleeding immediately. Then apply *Sheng Ji Jie Du Gao* (Engender Flesh, Resolve Toxins Paste) externally before bandaging. In critical cases, decoct the following in water, add 1 cup each of infant's urine and yellow wine (*i.e.*, rice wine), and take.

Radix Angelicae Sinensis (*Dang Gui*), 24g, Rhizoma Ligustici Wallichii (*Chuan Xiong*), 9g, Radix Rubrus Paeoniae Lactiflorae (*Chi Shao*), 2g, Gummum Olibani (*Ru Xiang*, vinegar processed), 6g, Myrrha (*Mo Yao*, vinegar processed), 6g, Flos Carthami Tinctorii (*Hong Hua*), 9g, Radix Rehmanniae (*Sheng Di*), 9g, Flos Lonicerae Japonicae (*Jin Yin Hua*), 15g, Fructus Forsythiae Suspensae (*Lian Cao*), 15g, raw Radix Glycyrrhizae (*Sheng Gan Cao*), 6g

In case of dry feces due to enduring disease, add Radix Et Rhizoma Rhei (*Da Huang*), 9g, and take 9g of Mirabilitum (*Mang Xiao*) separately.

54. *Shao Lin Ba Du Sheng Ji San* Shaolin Extract Toxins & Engender Flesh Powder

Ingredients: Radix Angelicae Dahuricae (*Bai Zhi*), 30g, Radix Trichosanthis Kirlowii (*Hua Fen*), 30g, Acacia Catechu (*Er Cha*), 30g, Gummum Olibani (*Ru Xiang*, vinegar processed) 15g, Myrrha (*Mo Yao*), 15g, Pyritum (*Zi Ran Tong*, dipped in vinegar 7 times), 30g, Calomelas (*Qing Fen*), 12g, Flos Lonicerae Japonicae (*Jin Yin Hua*), 18g, Fructus Forsythiae Suspensae (*Lian Qiao*), 18g, Cortex Phellodendri (*Huang Bai*), 18g, Rhizoma Coptidis Chinensis (*Huang*

Lian), 18g, Secretio Moschi Moschiferi (*She Xiang*), 6g, raw Radix Glycyrrhizae (*Sheng Gan Cao*), 12g

Method of preparation: First powder the Angelica, Trichosanthis, Lonicera, Forsythia, and Phellodendron. Then grind the Musk and the remaining 5 ingredients into a fine powder separately. Mix all the powders together and save in an air-tight bottle for use.

Method of use: In case of a shallow wound, just sprinkle the powder over the affected area and cover with white cloth. If the wound is deep, the powder can be made into a medicinal thread.[4] Then insert this into the base of the wound. If a scab has formed over the surface, mix the powder with roasted sesame oil (*Xiang You*) before applying to the affected area. Then cover with a cloth. Typically, this will cure the patient in from 3-5 days or not more than 7 days.

Commentary: This mixture has been a secret formula of the monk doctors of the Shaolin Monastery for generations. It is universally used for the treatment of failure to generate new tissue and enduring ulcers which will not close after injury.

55. Rx for the Treatment of Injury Due to Falling

Ingredients: Radix Angelicae Sinensis (*Dang Gui*), 15g, Rhizoma Ligustici Wallichii (*Chuan Xiong*), 9g, Flos Carthami Tinctorii (*Hong Hua*), 9g, Semen Pruni Persicae (*Tao Ren*), 9g, Radix Pseudoginseng (*San Qi,* powder and take separately), 3g, Radix Rubrus Paeoniae Lactiflorae (*Chi Shao*), 15g, Radix Rehmanniae (*Sheng Di*), 6g, Radix Saussureae Seu Vladimiriae (*Mu Xiang*), 1.5g

Decoct in water and take.

---

[4] *Yao Nian*, one of the classical methods of herbal medication

56. Rx for the Treatment of Blunt Injury to the Instep

Ingredients: Tabanus (*Meng Chong*), 5 bugs, Eupolyphaga Seu Opisthoplatia (*Tu Bie Chong*), 2 bugs, 2 snails (*Wo Niu*), Semen Pruni Persicae (*Tao Ren*), 9g, Gummum Olibani (*Ru Xiang*), 4.5g, Myrrha (*Mo Yao*), 4.5g

Grind the above 6 medicinals into powder. Mix this powder with raw honey (*Sheng Feng Mi*) before applying to the affected area. In case of skin rupture, the above ingredients should be mixed with some powdered Radix Pseudoginseng (*San Qi*) and carbonized powdered Radix Et Rhizoma Rhei (*Da Huang*) in equal parts. Sprinkle over the affected area.

57. Rx for the Treatment of Failure to Recover after Arrow Injury

Ingredients: Flos Carthami Tinctorii (*Hong Hua*), 6g, Calomelas (*Qing Fen*), 1.5g, Resina Garciniae (*Teng Huang*), 6g, Realgar (*Xiong Huang*), 9g, Cortex Phellodendri (*Huang Bai*), 15g, powdered carbonized toad skin (*Ha Ma Pi Tan Fen*), 1.5g, Alum (*Bai Fan*), 6g, Smithsonitum (*Lu Gan Shi*), 3g, Borneol (*Bing Pian*), 1.5g

Grind the above 9 medicinals into powder. Keep in a tightly closed bottle for use. Before application of the powder, the wound should be washed with a light salt solution in order to remove necrotic tissue. Then sprinkle the powder over the affected area and cover with a cloth. Internal use strictly prohibited.

58. Rx for the Treatment of Shovel[5] Injury to the Shoulder

Ingredients: Gummum Olibani (*Ru Xiang*, vinegar processed), 6g, Myrrha (*Mo Yao*, vinegar processed), 6g, Radix Angelicae Sinensis (*Dang Gui*), 9g, Squama Manitis Pentadactylis (*Chuan Shan Jia*), 9g, Spina Gleditschiae Chinensis (*Zao Jiao Ci*), 6g, Cortex Phellodendri (*Huang Bai*), 6g, Flos Lonicerae Japonicae (*Jin Yin Hua*), 6g, Fructus Forsythiae Suspensae (*Lian Qiao*), 6g, Bulbus Fritillariae Thunbergi (*Zhe Bei Mu*), 6g, Radix Angelicae Dahuricae (*Bai Zhi*), 6g, raw Radix Glycyrrhizae (*Sheng Gan Cao*), 6g, Herba Cum Radice Violae Yedoensis (*Di Ding*), 6g

Decoct in water and take with 30ml yellow wine (*i.e.*, rice wine).

59. Rx for the Treatment of Injury to the Bone Due to Poisonous Arrow

First take Semen Crotonis Tiglii (*Ba Dou*, remove the oil), 1 piece, live scarab beetle (*Qiang Lang*, remove head & feet), 1 bug, Semen Pruni Armeniacae (*Xing Ren*), 6 kernels, Semen Pruni Persicae (*Tao Ren*), 5 kernels.

Smash the above 4 medicinals into a paste and apply to the affected area. When local itching is felt, remove the paste and suck out the poisonous fluid by using cupping jars. The affected area should be washed 1-2 times with a salt solution before applying *Shao Lin Yuan Ming San* (Shaolin Original Brightness Powder). The next day, dress

---

[5] Shovel injury may mean being hit by a shovel, a traditional Chinese weapon, for instance carried by Friar Sandy in *A Journey to the West*. It may also refer to a tripping/tackling maneuver of that name which could easily result in falling on one's shoulder with the weight of one's own and possibly even the opponent's body.

the area with *Shao Lin Hong Yuan San* (Shaolin Red Origin Powder) and cover with white gauze. The addition of 3-5 *ji* of *Shaolin Yu Gu Tang* (Shaolin Bone Healing Decoction) will cure the patient.

60. *Shao Lin Yuan Ming San*
Shaolin Original Brightness Powder

Ingredients: Secretio Moschi Moschiferi (*She Xiang*), 0.3g, Alum (*Bai Fan*), 0.6g, Realgar (*Xiong Huang*), 9g, Radix Pseudoginseng (*San Qi*), 6g, Radix Angelicae Dahuricae (*Bai Zhi*), 9g

Grind the above medicinals into powder. This powder is indicated for the treatment of injuries due to broadsword, arrow, and spear.

61. *Shao Lin Hong Yuan San*
Shaolin Red Origin Powder

Ingredients: Flos Carthami Tinctorii (*Hong Hua*), 6g, Secretio Moschi Moschiferi (*Hong Hua*), 0.3g, Borneol (*Bing Pian*), 0.6g, Gummum Olibani (*Ru Xiang*, remove the oil), 3g, Myrrha (*Mo Yao*, remove the oil), 3g, Radix Angelicae Dahuricae (*Bai Zhi*), 6g, Radix Trichosanthis Kirlowii (*Tian Hua Fen*), 9g

Grind the above medicinals into a fine powder and store for use in a tightly closed bottle. This powder disperses inflammation and stops pain, resolves toxins and restrains and constrains.

62. *Shao Lin Yu Gu Tang*
Shaolin Bone Healing Decoction

Ingredients: Radix Angelicae Sinensis (*Dang Gui*), 24g, Rhizoma Ligustici Wallichii (*Chuan Xiong*), 9g, Flos Lonicerae Japonicae (*Jin Yin Hua*), 4.5g, Radix Angelicae Dahuricae (*Bai Zhi*), 9g, Radix Trichosanthis Kirlowii (*Tian Hua Fen*), 30g, Herba Mercurialis

Leiocarpae (*Tou Gu Cao*), 15g, raw Radix Glycyrrhizae (*Sheng Gan Cao*), 3g

Decoct in water and take. This formula is used in the treatment of enduring ulcers and suppurative conditions due to puncture wound by poisonous metal weapon.

63. *Shao Lin Jin Shang Zhi Fa*
Shaolin Metal Injury Treatment Method

Injury by metal weapons harms the flesh, blood, and qi. These three injuries carry toxins. If the blood is injured, then blood toxins will circulate all over the body. Since blood is stored in the liver, eventually the liver will become involved.

Method of treatment: "Absorb the toxins by hand," *i.e.*, use a jar to suck out the toxic juice. Then wash the affected area with aged salt and Radix Glycyrrhizae (*Gan Cao*) solution. Then sprinkle *Yu Jiang San* (Healing & Caring Powder) over the affected area and cover with white gauze.

64. *Jin Shang Yu Ling Dan*
Metal Injury Miraculous Recovery Elixir

Ingredients: Radix Angelicae Sinensis (*Dang Gui*), 9g, Rhizoma Ligustici Wallichii (*Chuan Xiong*), 9g, Pyritum (*Zi Ran Tong*, dipped in vinegar 7 times), 15g, Myrrha (*Mo Yao*, vinegar processed), 6g, Gummum Olibani (*Ru Xiang*, vinegar processed), 6g, Os Leopardis (*Bao Gu*), 6g, Lignum Sappanis (*Su Mu*), 9g, Eupolyphaga Seu Opisthoplatia (*Tu Bie Chong*), 9g, Squama Manitis Pentadactylis (*Chuan Shan Jia*), 6g, raw Radix Glycyrrhizae (*Sheng Gan Cao*), 6g,

Secret Shaolin Formulas

Tabanus (*Meng Chong*), 4.5g, *Shi Xiao San* (Loss of Smile Powder[6]), 15g

Method of preparation: Grind the above 12 medicinals into a fine powder and mix with *Shi Xiao San*. Then mix this with 300g of honey (*Feng Mi*) and some water in which rice has been washed. Make into pills the size of a pea. Store in a box ready for use and seal the lid with wax.

Method of administration: Take 5-7 pills per time with 30ml of yellow wine (*i.e.*, rice wine).

Functions: Resolves toxins and eliminates necrosis, disperses swelling and stops pain, engenders (new) flesh and restrains and constrains.

Mainly used in the treatment of enduring ulcers due to toxic swelling caused by all kinds of metal weapons.

65. Qi Wei Yu Jiang San
Seven Flavors Recover & Recuperate Powder

Ingredients: Secretio Moschi Moschiferi (*She Xiang*), 0.3g, Calomelas (*Qing Fen*), 0.6g, Alum (*Bai Fan*), 6g, Minium (*Huang Dan*), 6g, Resina Pini (*Song Xiang*), 6g, Radix Scutellariae Baicalensis (*Huang Qin*), 6g, Borneol (*Bing Pian*), 0.6g

Grind the above 7 ingredients into a fine powder. Mix well before placing in a tightly sealed bottle. In case of wound caused by metal weapon, wash the wound first with a solution of salt (*Yan*) and Radix Glycyrrhizae (*Gan Cao*). Afterward, sprinkle this powder over the

---

[6] See footnote #1 above, this chapter.

Fall, Strike, Bruise & Contusion Formulas

affected area and cover with white gauze. On the following day, apply *Shao Lin Ti Du Gao* (Shaolin Pull Out Toxin Plaster) locally.

66. *Shao Lin Ti Du Gao*
Shaolin Pull Out Toxins Plaster

Ingredients: Flos Lonicerae Japonicae (*Jin Yin Hua*), 15g, Secretio Moschi Moschiferi (*She Xiang*), 0.3g, Resina Pini (*Song Xiang*), 6g, Mercuric Oxide (*Hong Fen*), 15g, Gummum Olibani (*Ru Xiang*, remove the oil), 4.5g, Myrrha (*Mo Yao*, remove the oil), 4.5g, Pyritum (*Zi Ran Tong*, dipped in vinegar 7 times), 6g, Realgar (*Xiong Huang*), 4.5g, Borneol (*Bing Pian*), 0.9g

Method of preparation: First grind the herbs into powder. Then grind the rest of the ingredients also into powder and mix all of these powders together well. Add roasted sesame oil (*Xiang You*) and mix into a paste. Store for use in a tightly sealed porcelain jar.

Method of use: The wound should be washed with a salt solution and then this paste should be applied to the affected area. Cover with white gauze and change the dressing every day.

Functions: Resolves toxins, stops pain, dispels stasis, engenders flesh.

This plaster is universally used in the treatment of toxic skin lesions, ulceration, pus, and serous discharge and for long-term failure of astringency or localized redness, swelling, and pain due to blood stasis.

Commentary: This is an empirical formula created by the present abbot, De Chan, who presides over all the affairs of Shaolin Monastery. The number of patients cured by him with this prescription is over 1,000.

67. Shao Lin Qu Du Tang
Shaolin Expelling Toxins Decoction

Ingredients: Gummum Olibani (*Ru Xiang*, vinegar processed), 4.5g, Myrrha (*Mo Yao*, vinegar processed), 4.5g, Squama Manitis Pentadactylis (*Chuan Shan Jia*), 9g, Herba Cum Radice Taraxaci Mongolici (*Pu Gong Ying*), 30g, Flos Lonicerae Japonicae (*Jin Yin Hua*), 15g, Cortex Phellodendri (*Huang Bai*), 9g, Cortex Radicis Moutan (*Dan Pi*), 12g, Radix Scrophulariae Ningpoensis (*Xuan Shen*), 9g, Fructus Forsythiae Suspensae (*Lian Qiao*), 15g, Flos Chrysanthemi Indici (*Ye Ju Hua*), 30g, Radix Rubrus Paeoniae Lactiflorae (*Chi Shao*), 15g, Spina Gleditschiae Chinensis (*Zao Jiao Ci*), 9g, raw Radix Glycyrrhizae (*Sheng Gan Cao*), 6g

Decoct with water and take. Each day 1 *ji*. Take for 3-5 days consecutively. If taken with yellow wine (*i.e.*, rice wine), the effect will be better.

68. Shao Lin Gong Du San
Shaolin Attack Toxins Powder

Ingredients: Flos Lonicerae Japonicae (*Jin Yin Hua*), Fructus Forsythiae Suspensae (*Lian Qiao*), Semen Phaseoli Mungonis (*Lu Dou*, *i.e.*, mung beans), Cortex Phellodendri (*Huang Bai*), Sichuan Rhizoma Coptidis (*Chuan Huang Lian*), Cortex Radicis Moutan (*Mu Dan Pi*), Acacia Catechu (*Er Cha*), raw Radix Glycyrrhizae (*Sheng Gan Cao*), each in equal parts

Grind the above ingredients into powder. Take 15-30g with 30g yellow wine (*i.e.*, rice wine). Indicated for eruption of toxins from a wound.

69. Shang Jin Dong Gu Wan
Injured Sinews Remove the Bone Pills

Ingredients: Secretio Moschi Moschiferi (*She Xiang*), 1.5g, Semen Strychnotis (*Ma Qian Zi*, fry in oil & remove the hairs), 120g, Flos Carthami Tinctorii (*Hong Hua*), 150g, Semen Pruni Persicae (*Tao Ren*), 120g, Myrrha (*Mo Yao*, vinegar processed & remove the oil), 120g, Gummum Olibani (*Ru Xiang*, vinegar processed & remove the oil), 120g, Eupolyphaga Seu Opisthoplatia (*Tu Bie Chong*), 60g, Herba Ephedrae (*Ma Huang*), 90g, Semen Sinapis Albae (*Bai Jie Zi*), 60g, Radix Angelicae Sinensis (*Dang Gui*), 90g, Rhizoma Ligustici Wallichii (*Chuan Xiong*), 90g, Pyritum (*Zi Ran Tong*, dipped in vinegar 7 times), 90g, raw Radix Glycyrrhizae (*Sheng Gan Cao*), 60g

Method of preparation: Grind the Musk separately into a fine powder. Then grind the other 12 ingredients into powder and mix with the Musk. Boil 1000g of honey in a ceramic pot until the yellowish foam disappears. Strain this and mix with the herbal powder while still hot. The pills should weigh 6g each. Wrap in waxed paper. These pills should be kept in a kind of waxed pipe. Store for use in a cool, well ventilated place.

Method of administration: Take 1 pill with yellow wine (*i.e.*, rice wine) each time, 2 times per day.

Functions: Soothes the sinews and quickens the blood, frees the flow of the channels, quickens the network vessels, disperses swelling and stops pain, resolves toxins and transforms stasis

Commentary: These pills are quite effective for all cases of injury due to contusion and hit. They are prohibited during pregnancy.

70. Fei Long Duo Ming Dan
Flying Dragon Life-robbing Elixir

Ingredients: Borax (*Peng Sha*), 24g, Eupolyphaga Seu Opisthoplatia (*Tu Bie Chong*), 24g, Pyritum (*Zi Ran Tong*, dipped in vinegar 7 times), 24g, Sanguis Draconis (*Xue Jie*), 24g, Radix Saussureae Seu Vladimiriae (*Mu Xiang*), 18g, Radix Angelicae Sinensis (*Dang Gui*), 15g, Semen Pruni Persicae (*Tao Ren*), 9g, Rhizoma Atractylodis Macrocephalae (*Bai Zhu*), 15g, Cortex Radicis Acanthopanacis (*Wu Jia Pi*, wine processed), 15g, monkey bone (*Hou Gu*, vinegar processed), 15g, Rhizoma Corydalis Yanhusuo (*Yan Hu Suo*, wine stir-fried), 12g, Rhizoma Sparganii (*San Leng*, wine stir-fried), 12g, Lignum Sappanis (*Su Mu*), 12g, Feces Trogopterori Seu Pteromi (*Wu ling Zhi*, wine stir-fried), 9g, Radix Rubrus Paeoniae Lactiflorae (*Chi Shao*), 9g, Semen Allii Fistulosi (*Jiu Cai Zi*), 9g, raw Pollen Typhae (*Sheng Pu Huang*), 9g, processed Radix Rehmanniae (*Shu Di*), 9g, Cortex Cinnamomi (*Rou Gui*), 9g, Fructus Psoraleae Corylifoliae (*Bu Gu Zhi*, salt stir-fried), 9g, Guangdong Pericarpium Citri Reticulatae (*Guang Chen Pi*, stir-fried), 9g, Bulbus Fritillariae Cirrhosae (*Chuan Bei Mu*), 9g, Cinnabar (*Zhu Sha*), 9g, Radix Puerariae Lobatae (*Ge Gen*, stir-fried), 9g, Ramus Loranthi Seu Visci (*Sang Ji Sheng*), 9g, Radix Linderae Strychnifoliae (*Wu Yao*), 6g, Radix Et Rhizoma Notopterygii (*Qiang Huo*), 6g, Secretio Moschi Moschiferi (*She Xiang*), 1.5g, Cortex Eucommiae Ulmoidis (*Du Zhong*, salt & water stir-fried), 6g, Radix Gentianae Macrophyllae (*Jin Qiao*, stir-fried), 6g, Radix Peucedani (*Qian Hu*, stir-fried), 6g, scarab larvae (*Qi Cao*), 6g, Pericarpium Viridis Citri Reticulatae (*Qing Pi*, vinegar stir-fried), 6g

Method of preparation: Of the above 33 ingredients, first powder separately the Musk, Borax, Sanguis Draconis, and Pyritum. Then powder the other 29 herbal ingredients. Mix these two groups of powders together. After that, add 120g of cooked powdered glutinous

Fall, Strike, Bruise & Contusion Formulas

millet and make pills the size of peas. Dry and store in an air-tight container.

Method of administration: Take 9 grams each time, 3 times per day with yellow wine (*i.e.*, rice wine).

Functions: Quickens the blood and dispels stasis, frees the flow of the channels and quickens the network vessels, disperses swelling and stops pain, soothes the sinews and strengthens the bones

These pills are indicated for the treatment of all injuries due to fall and hit, pernicious ulcerations, injury to the sinews and fractures, pain in the waist and thigh due to wind damp evils, hemiplegia, and numbness of the four limbs. Their effect is quite good.

Commentary: This pill is also called *Shao Lin Fu Tong Dan* (Shaolin Buddha-freeing Elixir). It was created and kept secret by Fu Yu, abbot of the Shaolin Monastery in the Song Dynasty. It has been highly appreciated and has been passed down by generations of monk doctors and martial drillmasters. Approximately 3,000 cases treated by veteran monk doctor De Chan with this prescription have proven good results.

71. *Shao Lin Qi Li San*
Shaolin Seven *Li* Powder

Ingredients: Eupolyphaga Seu Opisthoplatia (*Tu Bie Chong*, remove head & legs), 24g, Sanguis Draconis (*Xue Jie*), 24g, Borax (*Peng Sha*), 24g, Rhizoma Atractylodis Macrocephalae (*Bai Zhu*, vinegar stir-fried), 15g, Semen Cuscutae (*Tu Si Zi*), 15g, Radix Saussureae Seu Vladimiriae (*Mu Xiang*), 15g, Feces Trogopterori Seu Pteromi (*Wu Ling Zhi*, wine processed), 15g, Guangdong Pericarpium Citri Reticulatae (*Guang Chen Pi*), 15g, raw Radix Et Rhizoma Rhei (*Sheng Da Huang*), 18g, scarab larvae (*Qi Cao*), 18g, Cinnabar (*Zhu*

Sha), 12g, monkey bone (*Hou Gu*), 12g, defatted Semen Crotonis Tiglii powder (*Ba Dou Shuang*), 9g, Rhizoma Sparganii (*San Leng*), 9g, Pericarpium Viridis Citri Reticulatae (*Qing Pi*), 9g, Radix Rubrus Paeoniae Lactiflorae (*Chi Shao*, vinegar stir-fried), 6g, Radix Linderae Strychnifoliae (*Wu Yao*), 6g, stir-fried Fructus Citri Seu Ponciri (*Zhi Qiao*), 6g, Radix Angelicae Sinensis (*Dang Gui*, wine stir-fried), 6g, raw Pollen Typhae (*Sheng Pu Huang*), 6g, stir-fried Pollen Typhae (*Chao Pu Huang*), 6g, Secretio Moschi Moschiferi (*She Xiang*), 4.5g

Method of preparation: First grind separately the Musk, Sanguis Draconis, defatted Semen Crotonis, Borax, and Cinnabar into a fine powder. Then grind and sieve the rest of the ingredients. Mix thoroughly both these two groups of powders. Put 0.2 grams in each packet, 12 packets to a box. Keep them in a dry, cool, well ventilated place until needed.

Method of administration: Take 1 or ½ packet each time. Or mix with vinegar into a paste and apply to the affected area. This powder is indicated for the treatment of pernicious skin lesions with suppurative toxins and unaccountable swellings and toxins. (This refers to all kinds of boils, furuncles, and carbuncles.)

Commentary: This formula has been proven efficacious in clinical practice for the foregoing symptoms by generations of monk doctors. It is one of the most common formulas used by the Patriarch De Chan.

72. *Shao Lin Shuang Jin Xu Gu Dan*
   Shaolin Strengthen Sinews & Connect the Bones Elixir

Ingredients: Radix Angelicae Sinensis (*Dang Gui*), 60g, Rhizoma Ligustici Wallichii (*Chuan Xiong*), 30g, Radix Albus Paeoniae Lactiflorae (*Bai Shao*), 30g, prepared Radix Rehmanniae (*Shu Di*),

Fall, Strike, Bruise & Contusion Formulas

30g, Cortex Eucommiae Ulmoidis (*Du Zhong*), 30g, Cortex Radicis Acanthopanacis (*Wu Jia Pi*), 60g, Rhizoma Drynariae (*Gu Sui Bu*), 90g, Ramulus Cinnamomi (*Gui Zhi*), 30g, Radix Pseudoginseng (*San Qi*), 30g, Os Tigridis (*Hu Gu*), 30g, Fructus Psoraleae Corylifoliae (*Bu Gu Zhi*), 60g, Semen Cuscutae (*Tu Si Zi*), 60g, Radix Codonopsis Pilosulae (*Dang Shen*), 60g, Fructus Chaenomelis Lagenariae (*Mu Gua*), 30g, Herba Artimisiae Anomalae (*Liu Ji Nu*), 60g, Eupolyphaga Seu Opisthoplatia (*Tu Bie Chong*), 90g, Radix Astragali Membranacei (*Huang Qi*), 30g, Radix Dipsaci (*Xu Duan*), 60g

Method of preparation: Grind the above 18 ingredients into a fine powder and sieve them. Take some sugar and make into sugar juice before sprinkling the medicinal powder with it. Shape this paste into pills the size of peas. Dry them in a cool place. Then store them in a bottle for use.

Method of administration: Take 9-12g each time, 2 times per day with yellow wine (*i.e.*, rice wine).

Functions: Supplements the qi and nourishes the blood, strengthens the sinews and connects the bones, dispels stasis and quickens the network vessels, warms and supplements the kidney chambers (*i.e.*, the low back).

These pills are indicated for the treatment of failure to recover from long-standing fractures and injuries, qi and blood vacuity, dizziness and vertigo, atonic limbs, and pain of the lumbar region and thighs.

Commentary: For injury to the sinews and bones due to *chin na* (*i.e.*, grappling techniques) in which the solitary usage of washing prescriptions (*i.e.*, liniments) are not enough, taking the above prescription internally will achieve a better result.

Note: *Chin na* is a type of Shaolin martial arts.

73. Shu Jin Huo Luo Tang
Soothe the Sinews & Quicken the Network Vessels Decoction

Ingredients: Herba Seu Flos Schizonepetae Tenuifoliae (*Jing Jie Sui*), 6g, Radix Ledebouriellae Sesloidis (*Fang Feng*), 6g, Herba Mercurialis Leiocarpae (*Tou Gu Cao*), 15g, Radix Et Rhizoma Notopterygii (*Qiang Huo*), 3g, Radix Angelicae Pubescentis (*Du Huo*), 7.5g, Radix Platycodi Grandiflori (*Jie Geng*), 6g, Folium Artimisiae Argyii (*Ai Ye*) produced in Qi Lian Shan (*i.e.*, Ningxia or Gansu Provinces), 6g, Fructus Zanthoxyli Bungeani (*Chuan Jiao*), 6g, Radix Rubrus Paeoniae Lactiflorae (*Chi Shao*), 15g, Herba Achilleae Alpiniae (*Yi Zhi Hao*), 15g

Wash and smoke with a concentrated juice made from the above ingredients. Three days of treatment will cure the patient for mild injury and 9 days for severe conditions. Three times per day. This prescription is especially effective for the treatment of superficial bruises with swelling and insidious pain due to grappling or other causes.

Note: Contraindicated in cases of ruptured skin.

74. Shao Lin Dang Gui Yin
Shaolin *Dang Gui* Drink

Ingredients: Radix Angelicae Sinensis (*Dang Gui*), 24g, Flos Carthami Tinctorii (*Hong Hua*), 9g, Herba Lycopi Lucidi (*Ze Lan*), 24g, Cortex Radicis Moutan (*Dan Pi*), 9g, Semen Pruni Persicae (*Tao Ren*), 9g, Lignum Sappan (*Su Mu*), 6g

Decoct in 1000ml each of water and wine. Reduce to 500ml of medicinal juice. Take internally.

Fall, Strike, Bruise & Contusion Formulas

For injury to the head, add Radix Et Rhizoma Ligustici Chinensis (*Gao Ben*), 9g. For injury to the hand, add Ramulus Cinnamomi (*Gui Zhi*), 6g. For injury to the waist, add Cortex Eucommiae Ulmoidis (*Du Zhong*), 9g, Semen Sinapis Albae (*Bai Jie Zi*), 6g, and Radix Achyranthis Bidentatae (*Niu Xi*), 12g. Decoct in water and take. Good results.

Functions: Quickens the blood and dispels stasis, disperses swelling and stops pain

This decoction is indicated for all types of local redness, swelling, and pain due to external injury from all causes and internal stasis.

75. Shao Lin Da Li Wan
Shaolin Great Strength Pills

Ingredients: Fructus Tribuli Terrestris (*Bai Ji Li*, soaked in saltwater & stir-fried), oxhide gelatin (*Huang Yu Jiao*, stir-fried in clam shell powder), Radix Angelicae Sinensis (*Dang Gui*, wine stir-fried), Radix Rehmanniae (*Sheng Di*, wine soaked & steam processed), 500g each

Method of preparation: Grind the above 4 medicinals into a fine powder and mix with 200g honey. Make pills the size of small marbles each weighing 6g.

Method of administration: For adults, 2 pills 2 times per day

Functions: Supplements the blood and boosts the qi

These pills are indicated in the treatment of pernicious skin lesions and ulcerous conditions, qi and blood dual vacuity, sallow facial complexion, emaciation, flaccid limbs, shortness of breath, fatigue, dizziness, and blurring of vision due to injuries of fall and strike.

76. Shao Lin Ying Xiong Wan
Shaolin Heroes Pill

Ingredients: Fructus Tribuli Terrestris (*Bai Ji Li*), 250g, a section of ox heel tendon (*Niu Ban Jin*) 9cm long, Os Tigridis (*Hu Gu*), Semen Cucumis Melonis (*Gan Gua Zi*), Plastrum Testudinis (*Gui Ban*), Sclerotium Poriae Cocos (*Fu Ling*), Radix Angelicae Sinensis (*Dang Gui*), 60g each, Radix Dipsaci (*Xu Duan*), 90g, Cortex Eucommiae Ulmoidis (*Du Zhong*), 90g, Fructus Psoraleae Corylifoliae (*Bu Gu Zhi*), 60g, Pyritum (*Zi Ran Tong*, dipped in vinegar 7 times), 15g, Eupolyphaga Seu Opisthoplatia (*Tu Bie Chong*), 10 bugs, Cinnabar (*Zhu Sha*), 21g, Lumbricus (*Di Long*), 15g

Method of preparation: Grind the Cinnabar separately. The other ingredients may all be ground together. Use honey to make pills, each weighing 9g. Take a small amount of powdered Cinnabar and coat each pill before it is wrapped with waxed paper. Keep them in a cool, well ventilated, dry place until use.

Method of administration: 1 pill each time, 2 times per day. For the first 2 weeks, take them with salt solution. The next 2 weeks take them with yellow wine (*i.e.*, rice wine). One month's treatment will cure the patient.

Functions: Enriches the blood and supplements the kidneys, supplements the qi and fortifies the spleen, soothes the sinews and quickens the blood, resolves tetany

This pill is mainly used for the treatment of poor health due to external injury and protracted disease, dizziness due to kidney vacuity, trismus of the body and limbs, rigidity of the four limbs, and difficulty walking.

77. Shao Lin Huo Xue Dan
Shaolin Quicken the Blood Elixir

Ingredients: Flos Carthami Tinctorii (*Hong Hua*), 30g, Semen Pruni Persicae (*Tao Ren*), 21g, Gummum Olibani (*Ru Xiang*, vinegar processed), 15g, Myrrha (*Mo Yao*, vinegar processed), 15g, Sanguis Draconis (*Xue Jie*), 15g, Lignum Sappanis (*Su Mu*), 15g, Acacia Catechu (*Er Cha*), 30g, Radix Angelicae Sinensis tails (*Gui Wei*), 30g, Radix Rubrus Paeoniae Lactiflorae (*Chi Shao*), 30g, Rhizoma Corydalis Yanhusuo (*Yan Hu Suo*), 30g, Cinnabar (*Zhu Sha*), 30g, Radix Angelicae Dahuricae (*Bai Zhi*), 30g, Rhizoma Arisaematis (*Nan Xing*), 21g, raw Radix Glycyrrhizae (*Sheng Gan Cao*), 27g, big-headed Radix Pseudoginseng (*Da Tou San Qi*), 9g, Secretio Moschi Moschiferi (*She Xiang*), 30g, Borneol (*Bing Pian*), 6g

Method of preparation: Grind separately the Musk, Borneol, Cinnabar, and Sanguis Draconis into a fine powder before grinding the rest of the 13 ingredients. Mix thoroughly all these powders. Use 90g of yellow rice flour to make a paste. Mix the powdered medicine with the paste and shape into pills the size of peas. Dry them and keep them in an air-tight bottle until needed.

Method of administration: Take 3-5 pills each time, 2 times per day with yellow wine (*i.e.*, rice wine). Adjust the dosage for children. These pills can be reground into powder and made into a paste with vinegar for local application to the affected area.

Functions: Quickens the blood and dispels stasis, disperses swelling and stops pain

Indications: Localized redness, swelling, pain, and bleeding due to external injury and suppurative and ulcerous wounds due to metal weapons

Commentary: Satisfactory results can be obtained with this formula in the treatment of abdominal mass, insidious pain of the lower abdomen, and in patients with excess tension patterns.

78. Shao Lin Zhan Jin Dan
Shaolin Extend the Sinews Elixir

Ingredients: Radix Angelicae Sinensis (*Dang Gui*), 60g, Rhizoma Ligustici Wallichii (*Chuan Xiong*), 60g, Flos Carthami Tinctorii (*Hong Hua*), 45g, Semen Pruni Persicae (*Tao Ren*), 45g, Pyritum (*Zi Ran Tong*, dipped in vinegar 7 times), 90g, Eupolyphaga Seu Opisthoplatia (*Tu Bie Chong*), 60g, Semen Strychnotis (*Ma Qian Zi*, oil process & remove the hairs), 90g, Sanguis Draconis (*Xue Jie*), 90g, Rhizoma Curcumae (*Jiang Huang*), 30g, Radix Angelicae Dahuricae (*Bai Zhi*), 60g, Radix Saussureae Seu Vladimiriae (*Mu Xiang*), 30g, Pericarpium Citri Reticulatae (*Chen Pi*), 30g, Lignum Aquilariae Agallochae (*Chen Xiang*), 15g, Fructus Foeniculi Vulgaris (*Xiao Hui Xiang*), 15g, Radix Pseudoginseng (*San Qi*), 60g, Gummum Olibani (*Ru Xiang*, vinegar processed), 90g, Myrrha (*Mo Yao*, vinegar processed), 90g, Radix Rubrus Paeoniae Lactiflorae (*Chi Shao*), 90g, Rhizoma Cyperi Rotundi (*Xiang Fu*, vinegar stir-fried), 90g, Acacia Catechu (*Er Cha*), 90g, Caulis Millettiae Seu Spatholobi (*Ji Xue Teng*), 12g, Secretio Moschi Moschiferi (*She Xiang*), 30g, Radix Aconiti (*Chuan Wu*, processed), 30g, Flos Impatientis Balsaminae (*Feng Xian Hua*), 60g, Herba Ephedrae (*Ma Huang*), 60g, Cinnabar (*Zhu Sha*), 9g, Borneol (*Bing Pian*), 3g

Method of preparation: Grind the Musk, Borneol, Sanguis Draconis, Cinnabar, Acacia, and Pyritum separately into a fine powder. Then grind the rest of the 21 medicinals. Boil some raw Licorice with spring water and use the resulting decoction to make pills the size of Chinese parasol tree seeds. Dry the pills in a cool place and keep them for use in a tightly sealed bottle.

Fall, Strike, Bruise & Contusion Formulas

Method of administration: For adults, take 4.5g each time, 2 times per day with yellow wine (*i.e.*, rice wine).

Functions: Soothes the sinews and quickens blood, disperses swelling and stops pain, resolves toxins and treats sores

These pills are indicated for the treatment of all kinds of injury due to fall and strike, pain due to blood stasis, injury of the sinews and bones, rigidity of the limbs and body, difficult movement, and pernicious ulcerous lesions with toxic pus.

Commentary: Prohibited to pregnant women.

79. Shao Lin Jiu Hu Dan
Shaolin Nine Tigers Elixir

Ingredients: Gummum Olibani (*Ru Xiang*, vinegar processed), 30g, Myrrha (*Mo Yao*, vinegar processed), 30g, Radix Angelicae Sinensis (*Dang Gui*), 150g, Rhizoma Ligustici Wallichii (*Chuan Xiong*), 90g, Rhizoma Arisaematis (*Nan Xing*, processed), 90g, Flos Carthami Tinctorii (*Hong Hua*), 90g, Radix Angelicae Dahuricae (*Bai Zhi*), 90g, Radix Ledebouriellae Sesloidis (*Fang Feng*), 90g, raw Radix Glycyrrhizae (*Sheng Gan Cao*), 60g

Method of preparation: Grind the above 9 ingredients into a fine powder. A dilute porridge is made out of an appropriate amount of yellow rice flour. Mix this together with the medicinal powder and make pills the size of peas. Keep these in a cool, well ventilated, dry place.

Method of administration: Take 9g each time, 2 times per day with yellow wine (*i.e.*, rice wine).

47

Functions: Quickens the blood and dispels stasis, disperses swelling and stops pain, expels pus and engenders flesh

Indications: Injuries caused by fall and strike, pain due to blood stasis, failure of relief of redness and swelling, sprain, spasm, and rigidity of the four limbs

Commentary: During the course of treatment, garlic and mutton are strictly prohibited. This formula is contraindicated for pregnant women. In case of pernicious skin ulceration with toxic pus, these pills can be reground into powder and mixed with vinegar to form a paste which can be applied to the affected area.

80. *Shao Lin Ping Feng Dan*
Shaolin Level Wind Elixir

Ingredients: Herba Cum Radice Asari (*Xi Xin*), 9g, raw Rhizoma Typhonii Gigantei Seu Radix Aconiti Coreani (*Sheng Bai Fu Zi*), 21g, Buthus Martensi (*Quan Chong*), 18g, Rhizoma Gastrodiae Elatae (*Tian Ma*), 18g, Radix Angelicae Dahuricae (*Bai Zhi*), 18g, raw Rhizoma Arisaematis (*Sheng Nan Xing*), 18g, Radix Et Rhizoma Notopterygii (*Qiang Huo*), 18g, Radix Ledebouriellae Sesloidis (*Fang Feng*), 21g, Margarita (*Zhen Zhu*, processed with beancurd), 0.6g, raw Radix Glycyrrhizae (*Sheng Gan Cao*), 30g

Method of preparation: Grind the Pearl separately into a fine powder before grinding the rest of the 9 medicinals. Mix these with the powdered Pearl. Use cold, boiled water to make pills the size of mung beans. Keep these in a bottle until needed.

Method of administration: Take 5-7 pills each time.

Functions: Eliminates wind and resolves tetany, resolves toxins and disperses swelling

Indications: Tetanus symptoms caused by injury due to fall and strike, such as opisthotonos, tremor, convulsions, lockjaw, and unconsciousness. It is also applicable for the treatment of redness and swelling due to metal wounds and ulcerous conditions with toxic pus.

81. *Shao Lin Ba Xian San*
Shaolin Eight Immortals Powder

Ingredients: Herba Verbenae (*Ma Deng Cao*), 15g, Semen Strychnotis (*Ma Qian Zi*, vinegar processed), 60g, Myrrha (*Mo Yao*, vinegar processed), 60g, Eupolyphaga Seu Opisthoplatia (*Tu Bie Chong*), 30g, Hirudo (*Shui Zhi*), 30g, Herba Ephedrae (*Ma Huang*), 45g, Borneol (*Bing Pian*), 3g

Method of preparation: First grind the Borneol into a fine powder before grinding the rest of the 7 medicinals. Mix thoroughly. Store in a tightly sealed bottle for use.

Method of use: Take internally 0.9-1g or sprinkle the powder directly on the wound. This powder can also be mixed into a paste for local application to the affected area.

Functions: Quickens the blood and breaks stasis, disperses swelling and stops pain, dispels wind and stops tetany

Indications: All kinds of injuries due to fall and strike, redness and pain, subdermal ecchymosis due to static blood, bone fractures, and injuries of the sinews, trismus due to tetanus, and a cold feeling in the legs due to wind damp, numbness of the joints, and paralysis of the limbs and body

Commentary: This prescription has been passed down from Shu Guang, the teacher of De Chan who is now the monk doctor of Shaolin Monastery. The Patriarch De Chan has used this prescription

Secret Shaolin Formulas

to achieve good results in 100 cases of injury due to fall and strike, sudden strain of the lumbar region, and localized redness and swelling.

82. *Shao Lin San Xian San*
Shaolin Three Immortals Powder

Ingredients: Raw Radix Glycyrrhizae (*Sheng Gan Cao*, remove the outer skin), 60g, Sichuan Rhizoma Coptidis (*Chuan Huang Lian*), 60g, Borneol (*Bing Pian*), 3g

Method of preparation: Grind the Borneol separately into powder before grinding the raw Licorice and Coptis.

Method of use: Take internally 3-4.5g. It can also be mixed with vinegar and then applied as a paste to the affected area. Good results.

Functions: Clears heat and resolves toxins, disperses swelling and stops pain

Indications: Ulceration and erosion of toxic skin lesions which are productive of pus and serous fluid, localized redness, swelling, and pain, and various carbuncles, furuncles, and toxic boils

Commentary: This is an effective formula De Chan used in the treatment of failure to heal of long-standing external, superficial lesions.

83. *Shao Lin Dong Yong Xing Jun San*
Shaolin Winter-Time Troop Deployment Powder

Ingredients: Radix Angelicae Sinensis (*Dang Gui*), 30g, Rhizoma Ligustici Wallichii (*Chuan Xiong*), 30g, Herba Seu Flos Schizonepetae Tenuifoliae (*Jing Jie Sui*), 30g, Radix Ledebouriellae

Sesloidis (*Fang Feng*), 30g, Herba Ephedrae (*Ma Huang*), 15g, Radix Angelicae Dahuricae (*Bai Zhi*), 30g, Ramulus Cinnamomi (*Gui Zhi*), 21g, Radix Angelicae Pubescentis (*Du Huo*), 15g, Radix Et Rhizoma Notopterygii (*Qiang Huo*), 15g, Fructus Zanthoxyli Bungeani (*Chuan Jiao*), 4.5g, dried Rhizoma Zingiberis (*Gan Jiang*), 3g, Radix Glycyrrhizae (*Gan Cao*), 9g

Method of preparation: Grind the above 12 medicinals into a fine powder and mix thoroughly for use.

Method of administration: Take 1.5g each time, 2-3 times per day.

Functions: Scatters cold and dispels wind, soothes the sinews and stops pain

Indications: Aversion to cold and fever due to exposure to wind cold, headache and stuffy nose, pain all over the body, rigidity of the four limbs, and soreness and pain of the lumbar region and legs

84. *Shao Lin Yao Nian*
Shaolin Medicinal Thread

Ingredients: Radix Violae Yedoensis (*Di Ding Gen*), 30g, Herba Cum Radice Taraxaci Mongolici (*Pu Gong Ying*), 30g, Flos Lonicerae Japonicae (*Jin Yin Hua*), 24g, Gummum Olibani (*Ru Xiang*, remove the oil), 9g, Myrrha (*Mo Yao*, remove the oil), 9g, Acacia Catechu (*Er Cha*), 12g, Flos Carthami Tinctorii (*Hong Hua*), 9g, Calomelas (*Qing Fen*), 6g, Sanguis Draconis (*Xue Jie*), 24g, Borneol (*Bing Pian*), 3.6g, Secretio Moschi Moschiferi (*she Xiang*), 1.5g

Method of preparation: Grind the herbal ingredients first and sieve them. Then grind the other ingredients separately. Mix thoroughly. Then make small rolls of the finest quality tissue paper into 1.5cm,

Secret Shaolin Formulas

2.1cm, and 3cm lengths packed with medicinal powder. Close both ends. Fill these medicinal threads with different amounts of medicinal powder in order to make different sized threads suitable for the treatment of different sized lesions. Pack in a box and seal with wax to store until needed.

Method of use: Clean away any pus and serous fluid with salt solution several times. Then insert the medicinal thread into the wound. Three to 5 rolls are 1 course of treatment. Change the dressing every 3 days. In most cases, 3 treatments will evacuate the pus and trigger the growth of new tissue. Seven treatments will heal the wound.

Functions: Resolves toxins and dispels necrosis, disperses swelling and stops pain, engenders flesh and grows muscle

Indications: Suppurative conditions, ulcers producing serous fluid, a cyanotic wound which fails to heal for a long time all due to injury by metal weapons

Commentary: This is an effective medicinal thread which has been used by the monk doctors of Shaolin Monastery for generations for the treatment of various pernicious, ulcerous, and suppurative lesions. Abbot De Chan has achieved remarkable results with this formula in the treatment of over 5,000 cases.

85. *Shao Lin Ba Zhen Dan*
Shaolin Eight Battle Formations Elixir

Ingredients: Radix Angelicae Sinensis (*Dang Gui*), 30g, Semen Pruni Persicae (*Tao Ren*), 30g, Gummum Olibani (*Ru Xiang*, vinegar processed), 15g, Myrrha (*Mo Yao*, vinegar processed), 15g, Sanguis Draconis (*Xue Jie*), 12g, Flos Lonicerae Japonicae (*Jin Yin Hua*),

21g, Squama Manitis Pentadactylis (*Chuan Shan Jia*), 9g, Pyritum (*Zi Ran Tong*, dipped in vinegar 7 times), 6g, Cortex Radicis Moutan (*Dan Pi*), 18g, Radix Angelicae Dahuricae (*Bai Zhi*), 12g, Sichuan Rhizoma Coptidis (*Chuan Huang Lian*), 12g, Radix Albus Paeoniae Lactiflorae (*Bai Shao*), 18g, Herba Cirsii Japonici & Herba Cephalanoplos Segeti (*Da Xiao Ji*), 15g each, Fructus Citri Seu Ponciri (*Zhi Qiao*), 12g, Guangdong Radix Saussureae Seu Vladimiriae (*Guang Mu Xiang*), 6g, Flos Caryophylli (*Ding Xiang*), 3g, raw Radix Glycyrrhizae (*Sheng Gan Cao*), 12g

Method of preparation: Grind the above 18 medicinals into a fine powder. Use the water in which rice has been washed to mix with this powder and make pills the size of peas. Dry them in the shade.

Method of administration: Take 1-3g each time, 2 times per day with yellow wine (*i.e.*, rice wine).

Functions: Breaks stasis and softens the hard, rectifies the qi and stops pain, resolves toxins, expels pus and engenders the flesh

Indications: All kinds of injuries due to fall and strike, pain due to blood stasis, ruptured or unruptured pernicious skin lesions, or toxic boils of all kinds and the failure of the wound to heal for a long time

Commentary: It is told that a martial monk by the name of Yue Neng of the Ming Dynasty set up a *ba gua zhen* (eight trigrams array) in a battle when he led a group of monks in the south. He was struck down by the outnumbering enemy and lost consciousness. He was taken for dead and the enemy left him alone. After the enemy had left, he regained consciousness and took this *hu shen dan* (*i.e.*, special elixir for critical conditions) which he always carried with him. He thereupon was able to leave the battlefield in 4 hours. Three days later, he had completely recovered. Hence the name *Ba Zhen Dan*.

86. Wu Sheng Ma Zui San
Five Raw Anesthetics Powder

Ingredients: Raw Radix Aconiti (*Sheng Cao Wu*), raw Rhizoma Arisaematis (*Sheng Nan Xing*), raw Rhizoma Pinelliae Ternatae (*Sheng Ban Xia*), raw Radix Aconiti (*Sheng Chuan Wu*), raw Radix Glycyrrhizae (*Sheng Gan Cao*), 60g each, Secretio Bufonis (*Chan Su*), 24g, Herba Cum Radice Asari (*Xi Xin*), 24g, Fructus Piperis Albi (*Bai Hu Jiao*), 60g, Flos Daturae (*Yang Jin Hua*), 30g

Method of preparation: Grind the herbs into powder.

Method of use: Make the powder into a paste and spread it over the area to be operated on.

Commentary: This prescription is widely used in monasteries. It serves as an anesthetic in cases which require surgical treatment of external injuries and toxic ulcers.

87. Shao Lin Jie Gu Dan
Shaolin Connect the Bones Elixir

Ingredients: Radix Angelicae Sinensis (*Dang Gui*), 30g, Radix Rehmanniae (*Sheng Di*), 30g, Radix Rubrus Paeoniae Lactiflorae (*Chi Shao*), 30g, Cortex Radicis Moutan (*Dan Pi*), 18g, goat hooves (*Yang Ti*), 30g, Radix Et Rhizoma Rhei (*Da Huang*), 30g, Cortex Phellodendri (*Huang Bai*), 30g, scarab larvae (*Qi Cao*), 30 pieces, earth louse (*Tu Shi, i.e.,* bedbugs), 100 pieces, Herba Mercurialis Leiocarpae (*Tou Gu Cao*), 60g, Pyritum (*Zi Ran Tong*, dipped in vinegar 7 times), 30g, Secretio Moschi Moschiferi (*She Xiang*), 3g

Method of preparation: Grind the Musk separately. Clean the scarab larvae before smashing them. Smash the bedbugs. Then grind the rest of the medicinals into powder and mix them thoroughly. Decoct 30g

Fall, Strike, Bruise & Contusion Formulas

of Flos Carthami Tinctorii (*Hong Hua*) with equal parts wine and water. Mix the resulting liquid after cooling with the medicinal powder and make pills the size of mung beans. Dry them in the shade before use.

Method of administration: Take 2-3g each time, 2 times per day.

Commentary: In case of acute bone fracture, first reduce and then immobilize with a splint. Then take these pills which will be effective.

88. *Jie Gu Tang*
Connect the Bones Decoction

Ingredients: Radix Angelicae Sinensis (*Dang Gui*), 9g, Flos Carthami Tinctorii (*Hong Hua*), 9g, Semen Pruni Persicae (*Tao Ren*), 9g, stir-fried Radix Et Rhizoma Rhei (*Da Huang*), 9g, Flos Chrysanthemi Indici (*Ye Ju Hua*), 30g, Cortex Radicis Moutan (*Dan Pi*), 12g, goat hooves (*Yang Ti*), 9g, Eupolyphaga Seu Opisthoplatia (*Tu Bie Chong*, remove the heads & legs), 6g, Pyritum (*Zi Ran Tong*, dipped in vinegar 7 times), 4.5g, raw Radix Glycyrrhizae (*Sheng Gan Cao*), 6g

Decoct in water and take.

89. *Shao Lin Shen Tong San*
Shaolin Spirit Connecting Powder

Ingredients: Gummum Olibani (*Ru Xiang*, vinegar process & remove the oil), 4.5g, Myrrha (*Mo Yao*, vinegar process & remove the oil), 4.5g, Sanguis Draconis (*Xue Jie*), 6g, Acacia Catechu (*Er Cha*), 6g, Radix Angelicae Dahuricae (*Bai Zhi*), 9g, Radix Trichosanthis Kirlowii (*Hua Fen*), 9g, (prepared) clear liquid feces (*Ren Zhong Huang*), 6g, Radix Pseudoginseng (*San Qi*), 6g, Borneol (*Bing Pian*), 3g

Method of preparation: Grind all the above medicinals into a powder for use.

Method of use: Take 1-2g each time, 2 times per day and chase with yellow wine (*i.e.*, rice wine) for adults. It should be used externally at the same time for better results. In case of ruptured skin, sprinkle the powder over the affected area. In cases where the skin is intact, make the powder into a paste with vinegar and apply it to the affected area. Both methods are quite effective.

Commentary: This is an empirical prescription created by Zhen Zhu, the abbot of the monastery. It is effective in the treatment of external injuries due to fall and strike and ulcerous lesions due to metal weapons.

90. Rx For the Treatment of *Jin Na Luo*[7] Injury of the Sinews & Bones

Ingredients: Secretio Moschi Moschiferi (*She Xiang*), 1.5g, Semen Strychnotis (*Ma Qian Zi*, stir-fry in oil & remove the hairs), 120g, Flos Carthami Tinctorii (*Hong Hua*), 150g, Semen Pruni Persicae (*Tao Ren*), 120g, Myrrha (*Mo Yao*, vinegar processed), 120g, Gummum Olibani (*Ru Xiang*, vinegar processed), 120g, Eupolyphaga Seu Opisthoplatia (*Tu Bie Chong*), 60g, Herba Ephedrae (*Ma Huang*), 90g, Semen Sinapis Albae (*Bai Jie Zi*), 60g, Radix Angelicae Sinensis (*Dang Gui*), 90g, Rhizoma Ligustici Wallichii (*Chuan Xiong*), 90g, Pyritum (*Zi Ran Tong*, dipped in vinegar 7 times), 90g, raw Radix Glycyrrhizae (*Sheng Gan Cao*), 60g

Method of preparation: Grind the Musk into a fine powder before grinding the rest of the medicinals which should also be sieved. Mix

---

[7] Literally, "tighten that gong." This may possibly be a type of weapon.

Fall, Strike, Bruise & Contusion Formulas

these with the Musk and shape into pills with 1030g of honey. Each pill should weigh 4.5g. Wrap them with waxed paper before packing them in a box for use.

Method of administration: Take 1 pill each time, 2 times per day. Chase with yellow wine (*i.e.*, rice wine).

Commentary: Quite effective for all kinds of external injury due to fall and strike. Prohibited to pregnant women.

91. *Wu Huang San*
Five Yellows Powder

Ingredients: Cortex Phellodendri (*Huang Bai*), 30g, Radix Scutellariae Baicalensis (*Huang Qin*), 30g, Rhizoma Coptidis Chinensis (*Huang Lian*), 30g, raw Pollen Typhae (*Sheng Pu Huang*), 30g, Radix Et Rhizoma Rhei (*Da Huang*), 30g, Radix Trichosanthis Kirlowii (*Tian Hua Fen*), 24g, raw Radix Glycyrrhizae (*Sheng Gan Cao*), 12g

Grind the medicinals into a fine powder and take 3-6g each time. This powder will achieve a good effect in all cases of ulcerous skin lesions.

Chapter Four

Shaolin Medicinal Wines

92. *Shao Lin Wu Xiang Jiu*
Shaolin Five Fragrances Wine

Ingredients: Flos Caryophylli (*Ding Xiang*), 9g, Radix Saussureae Seu Vladimiriae (*Mu Xiang*), 9g, Gummum Olibani (*Ru Xiang*, vinegar processed), 9g, Lignum Santali Albi (*Bai Tan Xiang*), 9g, Fructus Foeniculi Vulgaris (*Xiao Hui Xiang*), 9g, Radix Angelicae Sinensis (*Dang Gui*), 30g, Rhizoma Ligustici Wallichii (*Chuan Xiong*), 24g, Lignum Sappanis (*Su Mu*), 24g, Radix Achyranthis Bidentatae (*Niu Xi*), 24g, Flos Carthami Tinctorii (*Hong Hua*), 15g, good quality white alcohol (*Bai Jiu*), 500ml

Method of preparation: Crush the above ingredients and put them into a porcelain jar and cover with alcohol. Seal the lid of the jar with yellow earth and shake the jar 3 times per day. After 10 days, bury the jar 1 meter deep in the ground and cover with cut grass. After 30 days, remove from the earth and strain out the tincture. Wrap the dregs in gauze and squeeze out any remaining tincture. Rinse the dregs with fresh alcohol and mix this thoroughly with the tincture. Store in air-tight bottles.

Method of use: Apply topically to the affected area.

Functions: Quickens the blood and scatters stasis, disperses swelling and stops pain

Indications: Localized redness and swelling, fracture and dislocation, bruise and swelling of the skin, lumbar sprain, and *shan* qi

Note: Prohibited in cases where the skin is broken.

93. Bao Jiang Jiu
Protect the General Wine

Ingredients: Radix Angelicae Sinensis (*Dang Gui*), 60g, Rhizoma Ligustici Wallichii (*Chuan Xiong*), 24g, Lignum Sappanis (*Su Mu*), 24g, Flos Carthami Tinctorii (*Hong Hua*), 30g, Gummum Olibani (*Ru Xiang,* vinegar processed), 15g, Myrrha (*Mo Yao*, vinegar processed), 15g, Radix Angelicae (*Bai Zhi*), 15g, Ramulus Cinnamomi (*Gui Zhi*), 9g, Radix Astragali Membranacei (*Huang Qi*), 30g, Fructus Chaenomelis Lagenariae (*Mu Gua*), 24g, Radix Dipsaci (*Chuan Duan*), 15g, Ramus Loranthi Seu Visci (*Sang Ji Sheng*), 30g, Fructus Psoraleae Corylifoliae (*Bu Gu Zhi*), 15g, Cortex Radicis Mori Albi (*Sang Bai Pi*), 24g, prepared Radix Rehmanniae (*Shu Di*), 30g, Sichuan Tuber Curcumae (*Chuan Yu Jin*), 9g, Semen Pruni Persicae (*Tao Ren*), 30g, Radix Rubrus Paeoniae Lactiflorae (*Chi Shao*), 30g, Herba Mercurialis Leiocarpae (*Tou Gu Cao*), 30g, Cornu Cervi (*Lu Jiao*), 24g, Rhizoma Atractylodis Macrocephalae (*Bai Zhu*), 30g, Radix Pseudostellariae Heterophyllae (*Tai Zi Shen*), 15g, Radix Saussureae Seu Vladimiriae (*Mu Xiang*), 9g

Method of preparation: Crush the above ingredients into pieces and put them in a jar. Add 2740ml of the best quality white alcohol (*Bai Jiu*). The lid of the jar should be sealed with mud and straw. Keep the jar in a dry, well ventilated place. Shake it 3 times per day. The tincture is ready after 35 days. Strain the liquid and squeeze out the dregs by wrapping them in a white cloth. Stir the tincture thoroughly and keep under air-tight conditions.

Method of use: Take 30ml each time, 3 times per day. Drink a cup of warm water immediately after drinking the tincture to speed up its effect. Then rest in bed. If the local skin is not ruptured, this wine can be used to rub onto the affected area.

Functions: Quickens the blood and dispels stasis, dispels necrosis and engenders new (tissue), disperses swelling and stops pain, soothes the sinews and quickens the network vessels

Indications: Injury due to strike by fist and weapon, injury due to fall and strike, bruise and swelling due to blood stasis, bone fracture and injury of the sinews, pain in the waist and thighs

Note: This medicinal wine is quite effective not only in the treatment of disorders due to fall and strike but also in case of hemiplegia, paralysis, and numbness of the four limbs.

94. *Shao Lin Huo Long Jiu*
   Shaolin Live Dragon Wine

Ingredients: Live snakes (*Huo She*), 3 strips, Radix Angelicae Sinensis (*Dang Gui*), 60g, Flos Carthami Tinctorii (*Hong Hua*), 60g, prepared Radix Rehmanniae (*Shu Di*), 60g, Cortex Radicis Mori Albi (*Sang Bai Pi*), 60g, Radix Rubrus Paeoniae Lactiflorae (*Chi Shao*), 60g, Fructus Chaenomelis Lagenariae (*Mu Gua*), 60g, Radix Panacis Ginseng (*Song Shan Shen*, grown on Mt. Song [where the Shaolin Monastery is located]), 60g, Lignum Sappanis (*Su Mu*), 60g, processed Radix Aconiti (*Chuan Wu*), 30g, processed Radix Aconiti (*Cao Wu*), 30g, Caulis Millettiae Seu Spatholobi (*Ji Xue Teng*), 60g, Rhizoma Gastrodiae Elatae (*Tian Ma*), 60g, processed Rhizoma Pinelliae Ternatae (*Ban Xia*), 30g, Scolopendra Subspinipes (*Wu Gong*), 30 bugs, white alcohol (*Bai Jiu*), 6060ml

Method of preparation: Bind the heads of the snakes together with silk thread and also down the lengths of their bodies at three or four places. Pour the alcohol into a jar and drown the snakes in it by holding their heads beneath it before adding the other herbs. Seal the lid tightly. Shake the jar 3 times per day. After tincturing for 60 days, bury the jar 1 meter in the ground. Take out after another 40 days. Strain the medicinal liquid and squeeze out the dregs. Stir the liquid thoroughly and store in a tightly sealed container for use.

Method of administration: Take 15-20 ml each time, 3 times per day.

Functions: Quickens the blood and scatters stasis, disperses swelling and stops pain, soothes the sinews and opens the network vessels, settles tetany and dispels wind, supplements the blood and boosts the qi

Indications: Injury due to fall and strike, pain in the waist and thighs, numbness of the four limbs, and hemiplegia

95. *Luo Wang Zhu Gong Jiu*
Long-winded Emperor Assist Training Wine

Ingredients: Radix Rubrus Paeoniae Lactiflorae (*Chi Shao*), 1500g, Radix Angelicae Sinensis (*Dang Gui*), 1000g, Radix Rehmanniae (*Sheng Di*), 1500g, Rhizoma Ligustici Wallichii (*Chuan Xiong*), 1000g, Radix Achyranthis Bidentatae (*Niu Xi*), 1500g, Stamen Croci Sativi (*Zhang Hong Hua*), 90g, Fructus Chaenomelis Lagenariae (*Mu Gua*), 90g, Radix Saussureae Seu Vladimiriae (*Mu Xiang*), 90g, Ramulus Sophorae Japonicae (*Huai Zhi*), 60g, Pericarpium Citri Reticulatae (*Chen Pi*), 90g, Lignum Sappanis (*Su Mu*), 90g, Herba Mercurialis Leiocarpae (*Feng Xian Tou Gu Cao*), 60g, Ramulus Salicis Babylonicae (*Liu Zhi*), 60g, eagle claws (*Shan Ying Zhao*), 2 pairs, Bulbus Lilii (*Bai He*), 60g, Radix Astragali Membranacei

(*Huang Qi*), 1000g, Ramulus Pruni Persicae (*Tao Zhi*), 60g, white alcohol (*Bai Jiu*), 10 liters

Method of preparation: Crush the above ingredients into pieces and place them in a porcelain jar. Add 10 liters of alcohol and seal the lid with yellow earth. Bury the jar under the ground from 1—1½ meters deep. One hundred days later, unbury the jar. Strain out the liquid and squeeze out the dregs after wrapping in white cloth. Stir the liquid thoroughly. Strain the liquid repeatedly before decanting in 250ml bottles sealed with wax.

Method of administration: Take 15-30ml per time, 2-3 times per day.

Functions: Quickens the blood and transforms stasis, frees the channels and quickens the network vessels, scatters nodulation and stops pain, boosts the qi and strengthens the bones

Indications: Injury due to fall and strike, redness and swelling due to injury, pain due to blood stasis, numbness of the four limbs, hemiplegia, lack of strength of the entire body, shortness of breath, and fatigue

96. *Shao Lin Da Bu Jiu*
Shaolin Great Supplement Wine

Ingredients: Radix Angelicae Sinensis (*Dang Gui*), 30g, Rhizoma Ligustici Wallichii (*Chuan Xiong*), 30g, Fructus Chaenomelis Lagenariae (*Mu Gua*), 24g, Flos Carthami Tinctorii (*Hong Hua*), 24g, Radix Achyranthis Bidentatae (*Niu Xi*), 30g, Colla Cornu Cervi (*Lu Jiao Jiao*), 24g, Radix Astragali Membranacei (*Huang Qi*), 30g, Rhizoma Atractylodis Macrocephalae (*Bai Zhu*), 30g, Radix Codonopsis Pilosulae (*Dang Shen*), 30g, Ramulus Cinnamomi (*Gui Zhi*), 9g, Rhizoma Homalomenae (*Qian Nian Jian*), 9g, Radix Salviae

Miltiorrhizae (*Dan Shen*), 30g, Fructus Lycii Chinensis (*Qi Guo*), 15g, Radix Morindae Officinalis (*Ba Ji Tian*), 15g, Sclerotium Poriae Cocos (*Da Yun*), 15g, Herba Cynomorii Songarici (*Suo Yang*), 15g, prepared Radix Rehmanniae (*Shu Di*), 30g, snake from Mt. Qi Lian (*Qi Lian Shan She*), 15g, Hippocampus (*Hai Ma*), 15g, Carapax Amydae Sinensis (*Bie Jia*), 15g, Fructus Crataegi (*Shan Zha*), 30g, Fructus Germinatus Hordei Vulgaris (*Mai Ya*), 24g, Pericarpium Citri Reticulatae (*Chen Pi*), 15g, Cortex Cinnamomi (*Rou Gui*), 6g, Fructus Ligustri Lucidi (*Nu Zhen Zi*), 30g, Semen Cuscutae (*Tu Si Zi*), 24g, de-stemmed Radix Polygoni Multiflori (*He Shou Wu*), 30g, Bulbus Lilii (*Bai He*), 30g, Rhizoma Dioscoreae Hypoglaucae (*Bi Xie*), 15g, Fructus Tribuli Terrestris (*Bai Ji Li*), 15g, Radix Clematidis (*Wei Ling Xian*), 15g, processed Gummum Olibani (*Ru Xiang*), 9g, processed Myrrha (*Mo Yao*), 9g, Ramus Loranthi Seu Visci (*Sang Ji Sheng*), 24g, Caulis Polygoni Multiflori (*Ye Jiao Teng*), 15g, Caulis Millettiae Seu Spatholobi (*Ji Xue Teng*), 30g, Rhizoma Cimicifugae (*Sheng Ma*), 15g, Radix Anemarrhenae (*Zhi Mu*), 24g, Semen Gingkonis Bilobae (*Bai Guo*), 15g, Fructus Alpiniae Oxyphyllae (*Yi Zhi Ren*), 15g, Plastrum Testudinis (*Gui Ban*), 15g, white alcohol (*Bai Jiu*), 3 liters

Method of preparation: Chop the above 44 ingredients and put them in a porcelain jar. Add alcohol. Seal the lid well with yellow earth. Shake once per day. Strain out the liquid after tincturing for 3 months. Squeeze out the dregs by wrapping the herbs in white cloth. Stir thoroughly. Strain the liquid again through 3-5 layers of gauze into a porcelain jar and keep air-tight for use.

Method of administration: Take 15-20ml each time, 2 times per day internally.

Functions: Supplements the blood and boosts the qi, strengthens the low back and invigorates the kidneys, frees the channels and quickens the network vessels, opens the stomach and disperses food

Indications: Pallor, palpitations, shortness of breath, weakness of the four limbs, impeded movement of the joints, food stagnation, cold accumulation, qi accumulation, blood accumulation, cold limbs due to kidney vacuity, dizziness, blurred vision, clear, prolonged urination, loose stools, weakness due to protracted illness in turn due to either external or internal injury, paralysis, apoplexy, coma, hemiplegia, prolapse of central qi, and anal prolapse. If small doses are taken frequently, its revitalizing effect is conducive to longevity.

Commentary: Caution is advised in patients with hyperactivity of liver yang and blood vacuity due to internal heat and in those with heart problems.

97. *Shao Lin Yu Gong Jiu*
   Shaolin Abundant Justice Wine

Ingredients: Radix Codonopsis Pilosulae (*Dang Shen*), 90g, Radix Astragali Membranacei (*Huang Qi*), 500g, Radix Rehmanniae (*Sheng Di*), 180g, prepared Radix Rehmanniae (*Shu Di*), 180g, Fructus Corni Officinalis (*Shan Zhu Yu*), 180g, Cortex Eucommiae Ulmoidis (*Du Zhong*), 180g, Radix Angelicae Sinensis tails (*Gui Wei*), 180g, Radix Polygoni Multiflori (*He Shou Wu*), 250g, Bulbus Lilii (*Bai He*), 180g, Tuber Ophiopogonis Japonicae (*Mai Men Dong*), 180g, Semen Biotae Orientalis (*Bai Zi Ren*), 180g, Semen Coicis Lachryma-Jobi (*Yi Yi Ren*), 90g, Dens Draconis (*Long Chi*), 90g, Herba Dendrobii (*Shi Hu*), 90g, Radix Albus Paeoniae Lactiflorae (*Bai Shao*), 90g, Exocarpium Citri Grandis (*Ju Hong*), 90g, Fructus Lycii Chinensis (*Qi Guo*), 270g, Caulis Millettiae Seu Spatholobi (*Ji Xue Teng*), 270g, Semen Glycinis Hispidae (*Hei Dou, i.e.,* black soybeans), 180g, deer kidney (*Lu Shen*), 30g, dog kidney (*Gou Shen*), 30g, donkey kidney (*Lu Shen*), 30g, Placenta Hominis (*Zi He Che*), 90g, Ramulus Cinnamomi (*Gui Zhi*), 60g, Radix Praeparatus Aconiti Carmichaeli (*Fu Zi*), 30g, Cortex Cinnamomi (*Rou Gui*), 30g, Semen Cuscutae (*Tu Si Zi*), 250g, Fructus Alpiniae Oxyphyllae (*Yi Zhi Ren*),

210g, Fructus Crataegi (*Shan Zha*), 250g, Semen Pini (*Song Zi Ren*), 60g, Fructus Germinatus Hordei Vulgaris (*Mai Ya*), 210g, Herba Ecliptae Prostratae (*Han Lian Cao*), 210g, Arillus Euphoriae Longanae (*Long Yan Rou*), 210g, Buthus Martensi (*Quan Chong*), 60g, Scolopendra Subspinipes (*Wu Gong*), 30g, Radix Rubrus Paeoniae Lactiflorae (*Chi Shao*), 180g, Flos Carthami Tinctorii (*Hong Hua*), 60g, Rhizoma Gastrodiae Elatae (*Tian Ma*), 180g, Fructificatio Ganodermae Lucidae (*Ling Zhi Cao*), 120g, Fructificatio Tremellae (*Jin Er*), 60g, Semen Cassiae Torae (*Cao Jue Ming*), 120g, Flos Chrysanthemi Morifolii (*Ju Hua*), 120g, Rhizoma Atractylodis Macrocephalae (*Bai Zhu*), Flos Hibisci (*Mu Jin Hua*), 60g each, Herba Cum Radice Violae Yedoensis (*Di Ding*), 60g

Method of preparation: Crush the nuts first among the above 44 ingredients. Chop all the medicinals before placing them in a porcelain jar. Add 20 liters of best quality white alcohol (*Bai Jiu*) and seal the lid so that it is air-tight. Bury the jar from 1—1½ meters deep. Remove the jar after about 100 days. Strain the medicinal wine and squeeze out all the juice from the dregs by wrapping them in white gauze. Stir thoroughly and filter 3 times. Decant into 250ml bottles after it has become transparent. Store air-tight for use.

Method of administration: Take 15-20ml each time.

Functions: Supplements the qi and quickens the blood, boosts the liver and enriches the kidneys, blackens the hair and secures the teeth, removes pigmentation[1] and brightens the facial complexion, strengthens the sinews and bones. If taken frequently in small doses, it facilitates health and prevents disease for the purpose of regaining the vitality and achieving longevity.

---

[1] This probably refers to so-called liver spots or patches of skin discoloration associated with aging.

Indications: Sallow complexion, emaciation, dizziness, blurred vision, shortness of breath, palpitations, weakness of the four limbs, premature greying of the moustache and hair, balding due to blood vacuity, reduced auditory acuity, tinnitus, and loose teeth. In addition, this wine is effective for all chronic diseases.

Commentary: This prescription was created by Fu Yu, the great monk authorized by the emperor of the Song Dynasty. It has proven effective for supplementing the five viscera and for strengthening one's body, for preventing the debility of aging, and for achieving longevity.

Note: Care should be exercised in the usage of this wine in patients with heart disease, internal heat, or other exuberant evils.

Chapter Five

Shaolin Herbal Plasters

98. Ha Ma Pi Gao
Toad Skin Plaster

Ingredients: Toad skin (*Ha Ma Pi*), 30g, Squama Manitis Pentadactylis (*Chuan Shan Jia*), 30g, Pyritum (*Zi Ran Tong*, dipped in vinegar 7 times), 15g, Acacia Catechu (*Er Cha*), 15g, Cortex Phellodendri (*Huang Bai*), 15g, Radix Rumicis Madaionis (*Tu Da Huang*), 15g, Radix Angelicae (*Bai Zhi*), 15g, Calomelas (*Qing Fen*), 6g, Sanguis Draconis (*Xue Jie*), 6g, Borneol (*Bing Pian*), 3g

Method of preparation: Grind the above ingredients into a fine powder. Make into a paste by mixing in aged vinegar (*Chen Cu*). Store in a bottle for use.

Method of use: Apply paste to the affected area and change the dressing every day.

Functions: Resolves toxins and expels pus, softens the hard and breaks nodulation, quickens the blood and scatters stasis, disperses swelling and stops pain

Indications: Ulcerous conditions due to external injury with either ruptured or unruptured skin, suppurative osteomyelitis, carbuncle on the back of the neck, scrofula, multiple abscesses, common carbuncles, ganglion cysts, and pernicious skin lesions

Commentary: This is an effective prescription created by Shen Ju, a great monk of the late Qing Dynasty, based on his 30 years' experience in treating pernicious skin lesions and toxic pus. More than 3,000 patients have been cured by this prescription.

99. Shao Lin Hui Chun Gao
Shaolin Return Spring Plaster

Ingredients: Gummum Olibani (*Ru Xiang*), 30g, Myrrha (*Mo Yao*), 30g, Scolopendra Subspinipes (*Wu Gong*), 30g, Flos Lonicerae Japonicae (*Jin Yin Hua*), 150g, Fructus Forsythiae Suspensae (*Lian Qiao*), 150g, Herba Cum Radice Violae Yedoensis (*Di Ding*), 150g, Cortex Phellodendri (*Huang Bai*), 150g, Radix Angelicae (*Bai Zhi*), 150g, Radix Rubrus Paeoniae Lactiflorae (*Chi Shao*), 150g, Sclerotium Polypori Umbellati (*Zhu Ling*), 150g, Radix Angelicae Sinensis tails (*Gui Wei*), 150g, raw Radix Astragali Membranacei (*Sheng Huang Qi*), 150g, Rhizoma Ligustici Wallichii (*Chuan Xiong*), 90g, Radix Ampelopsis Japonicae (*Bai Lian*), 150g, Camphora (*Chang Nao*), 30g, Calomelas (*Qing Fen*), 30g, Mercuric Oxide (*Hong Fen*), 30g, Minium (*Guang Dan*), 90g, Sanguis Draconis (*Xue Jie*), 30g, Borneol (*Bing Pian*), 9g, raw Radix Glycyrrhizae (*Sheng Gan Cao*), 60g, roasted sesame oil (*Xiang You*), 12 kilograms, Squama Manitis Pentadactylis (*Chuan Shan Jia*), 150g, Acacia Catechu (*Er Cha*), 30g, Sichuan Rhizoma Coptidis Chinensis (*Chuan Huang Lian*), 150g, raw Fructus Gardeniae Jasminoidis (*Sheng Zhi Zi*), 150g

Method of preparation: Grind the Frankincense, Myrrh, Safflower, Calomelas, Camphora, Borneol, Acacia Catechu, and Sanguis Draconis into a fine powder, each separately. Add 12 kilograms of roasted sesame oil into a pot with the remaining 16 medicinals. Stir-fry these until they have become burnt using a moderate fire. Remove the dregs and filter the oil after it has cooled. Then reheat this medicated oil with a moderate fire until ripples move from the center of its surface to the outer margins of the pot and till the smoke turns from dark greenish black to white. At this point, the fire should be turned off and the powdered Minium should be added while stirring so as to prevent their lumping and settling to the bottom. Each 300 grams of medicated oil can be mixed with 110g of powdered minerals. This should continue until the contents are thoroughly mixed.

Remove the pot from the stove and pour the contents into cold water. Immerse the medicine in water for 10-15 days. Change the water 2 times per day to remove the fire toxins. Heat and soften this medicinal mass again and add the remaining 8 powdered ingredients. The plaster is ready when all the ingredients are thoroughly mixed.

Spreading the plaster: A piece of plaster 7.5cm in length should weigh 9g, and a piece 5cm long should weigh 5g. Seal and label for storage (indicating the measurement and date of preparation). Each box of 10 plasters should be tightly sealed.

Method of use: Clean the ulcerated area with a weak salt solution before applying the plaster. Change the plaster every 7 days.

Functions: Resolves toxins and treats sores, expels pus and eliminates necrosis, engenders the flesh, restrains and contains, disperses swelling and stops pain

Indications: Wounds due to metal weapons, pernicious ulcerous skin conditions producing toxic pus, redness, swelling, and pain, carbuncles and gangrene, carbuncles on the back of the neck, poisonous insect bites, etc.

Commentary: This is a secret formula passed down by Zhen Jun, a great monk of Shaolin Monastery. Abbot De Chan has treated over 1,000 cases with this prescription. Most often, just 1-2 applications will cure a wound. Three to 5 may be necessary in severe cases.

Itching around the edge of the plaster is a good sign that the plaster is working and it should therefore be kept in place.

100. *Shao Lin Qian Chui Gao*
Shaolin 1,000 Hammers Plaster

Ingredients: Semen Pruni Armeniacae (*Xing Ren*), 40 kernels, Semen Pruni Persicae (*Tao Ren*), 40 kernels, Fructus Crotonis Tiglii (*Ba Dou*), 7 pieces, aged Aerugo (*Chen Tong Lu, i.e.,* blue-green copper rust), 9g, Borneol (*Bing Pian*), 6g, roasted sesame oil (*Xiang You*)

Method of preparation: Crush the above 5 medicinals in a stone trough. Remove them and smash into a paste with a pestle. Add 60g of roasted sesame oil and mix thoroughly. Pour into a bottle and store air-tight for use.

Method of use: Apply to the affected area. Change the dressing every day.

Functions: Resolves toxins and softens the hard, disperses swelling and stops pain

Indications: Pernicious skin ulcers producing toxic pus, localized redness and swelling, carbuncles and gangrene, and mastitis

Commentary: Abbot De Chan has treated over 750 cases with this prescription who have witnessed its remarkable effect after its first external application.

101. *Shao Lin Wu Xian Gao*
Shaolin Five Immortals Plaster

Ingredients: Secretio Moschi Moschiferi (*She Xiang*), 0.6g, Sichuan Rhizoma Coptidis Chinensis (*Chuan Huang Lian*), 30g, raw Radix

Glycyrrhizae (*Sheng Gan Cao*), 60g, Minium (*Guang Dan*), 9g, Borneol (*Bing Pian*), 0.6g, fresh roasted sesame oil (*Sheng Xiang You*), 65g

Method of preparation: Grind the Coptis and raw Licorice into a fine powder. Then grind the Musk separately. Mix the resulting powders together until thoroughly blended and make them into a paste by adding the roasted sesame oil. Keep this paste air-tight in a porcelain jar until needed.

Method of use: In case of broken skin, clean the affected area with warm, boiled water. For those whose skin is not ruptured, wash and rub the affected area with an Alum (*Bai Fan*) solution before applying the plaster. Change the dressing every day.

Functions: Resolves toxins, disperses swelling, stops pain, engenders the flesh, and restrains and contains

Indications: Redness, swelling, and pain caused by carbuncles, gangrene, or boils of all kinds with ruptured or unruptured skin and production of pus and serous fluid and failure to form a scab for a prolonged period of time

Commentary: The great monk Zhen Zhu used this prescription in the treatment of carbuncles, gangrene, and boils of all kinds and pernicious skin ulcers in over 1,000 cases with good effect.

102. *Shao Lin Guan Yin Gao*
Shaolin Temple Music Plaster

Ingredients: Ramulus Cinnamomi (*Gui Zhi*), 60g, Ramulus Mori Albi (*Sang Zhi*), 30g, Flos Carthami Tinctorii (*Hong Hua*), 30g, Semen Pruni Persicae (*Tao Ren*), 90g, Gummum Olibani (*Ru Xiang*, vinegar process & remove the oil), 60g, Myrrha (*Mo Yao*, vinegar process &

remove the oil), 60g, Radix Trichosanthis Kirlowii (*Tian Hua Fen*), 60g, Radix Angelicae (*Bai Zhi*), 60g, Radix Et Rhizoma Rhei (*Da Huang*, wine processed), 60g, Radix Rubrus Paeoniae Lactiflorae (*Chi Shao*), 60g, Fructus Chaenomelis Lagenariae (*Mu Gua*), 60g, Lignum Sappanis (*Su Mu*), 30g, Radix Achyranthis Bidentatae (*Niu Xi*), 60g, Pyritum (*Zi Ran Tong*), 30g, Herba Ajugae (*Shu Jin Cao*), 30g, Cortex Radicis Moutan (*Mu Dan Pi*), 30g, Herba Artemisiae Anomalae (*Liu Ji Nu*), 60g, Caulis Akebiae Mutong (*Mu Tong*), 30g, Caulis Millettiae Seu Spatholobi (*Ji Xue Teng*), 60g, Rhizoma Corydalis Yanhusuo (*Yan Hu Suo*, vinegar processed), 60g, Acacia Catechu (*Er Cha*), 60g, Secretio Moschi Moschiferi (*She Xiang*), 15g, raw Radix Glycyrrhizae (*Sheng Gan Cao*), 30g, Minium (*Guang Dan*), 300g, Borneol (*Bing Pian*), 15g, Mercuric Oxide (*Hong Fen*), 30g, Radix Angelicae Sinensis (*Dang Gui*), 60g, Rhizoma Ligustici Wallichii (*Chuan Xiong*), 45g, Guangdong Radix Saussureae Seu Vladimiriae (*Guang Mu Xiang*), 30g, Calomelas (*Qing Fen*), 30g, roasted sesame oil (*Xiang You*), 2 kilograms

Method of preparation: Grind the Musk, Borneol, Calomelas, Mercuric Oxide, Acacia Catechu, Pyritum, Frankincense, Myrrh, and Minium separately into fine powders and reserve. Chop the rest of the ingredients and stir-fry in the oil until they are burnt. Remove the dregs and filter. Then reheat the oil over a moderate fire until ripples from the center move to the outer margins of the pot. (The following procedure is the same as in preparing *Shao Lin Hui Chun Gao*.) Add each of the above powders separately and blend them into the paste thoroughly.

Spreading the plasters: A plaster 8cm in length should weigh 9g. One 5cm long should weigh 4.5g. Mark the dimensions and date of preparation on each plaster and pack them in a box, 10 pieces each.

Method of use: Apply to the affected area.

Functions: Resolves toxins and scatters nodulations, quickens the blood and dispels stasis, disperses swelling and stops pain, connects the bones and reunites the sinews

Indications: All injuries due to fall and strike, pain due to blood stasis, pernicious skin ulcers producing toxic pus, ruptured or unruptured and failing to scab for a long time, dislocation, fracture, numbness of the four limbs, hemiplegia, pain of the waist and thighs, spasms or rigidity of the hands and feet, and difficulty walking

Commentary: This prescription has been passed down from Fu Ju, a great monk from the Shaolin Monastery of the Song Dynasty. Master Abbot Zhen Jun treated over 1,000 cases of the above complaints with this prescription with good result. Therefore, this plaster is well-known for 100 *li* surrounding the monastery and is also called *Shao Lin Shen Gao* (Shaolin Spirit Plaster).

103. *Shao Lin Bai Yi Pu Sa Gao*
Shaolin White-Coated Bodhisattva Plaster

Ingredients: Radix Angelicae Sinensis crowns (*Dang Gui Tou*), 30g, Radix Rubrus Paeoniae Lactiflorae (*Chi Shao*), Radix Albus Paeoniae Lactiflorae (*Bai Shao*), 30g each, Flos Carthami Tinctorii (*Hong Hua*) 30g, blackened Cortex Radicis Moutan (*Hei Mu Dan*), 30g, Gummum Olibani (*Ru Xiang*, vinegar processed), 45g, Myrrha (*Mo Yao*, vinegar processed), 45g, Squama Manitis Pentadactylis (*Chuan Shan Jia*), 45g, raw Concha Ostreae (*Sheng Mu Li*), 45g, Eupolyphaga Seu Opisthoplatia (*Tu Bie Chong*), 45g, Acacia Catechu (*Er Cha*), 45g, Guangdong Radix Saussureae Seu Vladimiriae (*Guang Mu Xiang*), 15g, Southern Flos Caryophylli (*Nan Ding Xiang*), 6g, Calomelas (*Qing Fen*), 30g, Mercuric Oxide (*Hong Fen*), 30g, raw Radix Glycyrrhizae (*Sheng Gan Cao*), 21g, Cortex Pruni Persicae (*Tao Shu Pi*), 60g, Ramulus Salycis (*Liu Shu Zhi*), 60g, Ramulus Cinnamomi (*Gui Zhi*), 30g, Secretio Moschi Moschiferi (*She Xiang*), 30g,

Minium (*Qian Dan*), 300g, Borneol (*Bing Pian*), 9g, roasted sesame oil (*Xiang You*), 1200g

Method of preparation: Of the above 22 medicinals, grind separately and reserve the Musk, Borneol, Mercuric Oxide, Minium, Acacia Catechu, Frankincense, and Myrrh. Crush the rest of the 15 ingredients before stir-frying them in the oil over a moderate fire until burnt. Filter the medicated oil and then reheat the oil until the smoke rising from it has turned from dense and greenish to white. Remove the oil from the fire when ripples spread out from the center and add the Minium (stirring constantly to avoid lumping and burning).

Pour the medicated oil into cold water in order to remove the fire toxins. The last step is to reheat the paste again and add the powdered Musk, Borneol, and other reserved ingredients. The plaster is ready when all the ingredients are thoroughly mixed.

Spreading the plasters: a plaster 9cm in length should weigh 9g. One 7cm long should weigh 6g, while one 5cm should weigh 3.5g. Pack 10 plasters to a box for use.

Method of use: Apply to the affected area.

Functions: Quickens the blood and dispels stasis, disperses swelling and stops pain, connects the bones and reunites the sinews

Indications: All kinds of injuries due to fall and strike, dislocation and fracture, sprain of the lumbar area due to unexpected fall and stumbling, swelling and pain due to blood stasis

Commentary: Abbot De Chan has treated over 600 cases of injury due to fall and strike, strain of the low back, *shan*, injury of the sinews, and bone fractures with this plaster. It is especially effective for relieving pain due to fall and strike injury and pain due to static blood.

104. *Shao Lin Yi Chuang Gao*
Shaolin Medical Ulcer Plaster

Ingredients: Calomelas (*Qing Fen*), 30g, Flos Lonicerae Japonicae (*Jin Yin Hua*), 60g, Acacia Catechu (*Er Cha*), 30g, Radix Angelicae (*Bai Zhi*), 60g, Cortex Phellodendri (*Huang Bai*), 60g, Radix Rumicis Madaionis (*Tu Da Huang*), 60g, Resina Garciniae (*Teng Huang*), 15g, prepared human feces (*Ren Chong Huang*), 60G, Gummum Olibani (*Ru Xiang*, remove the oil), 30g, Myrrha (*Mo Yao*, remove the oil), 30g, Borneol (*Bing Pian*), 15g, roasted sesame oil (*Xiang You*), 800g

Method of preparation: Grind all the above medicinals, except for the Calomelas and Borneol, into a fine powder and sieve it before adding the Calomelas and Borneol. Add the roasted sesame oil and mix into a paste. Store this paste in a porcelain jar for use.

Method of use: Apply to the affected area. Change the plaster every day.

Functions: Resolves toxins and eliminates necrosis, disperses swelling and stops pain

Indications: Ulcerous conditions resulting from metal weapons which are producing a toxic fluid with a repulsive odor, ruptured or unruptured carbuncles and gangrene, and pain due to unaccountable swelling

Commentary: This is a secret prescription kept by the great monk Zhen Zhu. Over 1,000 cases of pernicious ulcer with pus have been treated with this formula. Typically, 3-4 treatments will produce the desired effect.

105. *Wu Zhi Gao*
Five Twigs Plaster

Ingredients: Ramulus Pruni Persicae (*Tao Shu Zhi*), Ramulus Sophorae Japonicae (*Huai Zhi*), Ramulus Salicis (*Liu Shu Zhi*), Ramulus Populi Suaveolentis (*Qing Yang Shu Zhi*), Ramulus Ponciri Trifoliati (*Gou Shu Zhi*), 2500g each (fresh ones are preferable), Squama Manitis Pentadactylis (*Chuan Shan Jia*), 100g, fresh Folium Cannabis Sativae (*Xian Ma Ye*), 1500g, tender Pericarpium Fructi Juglandis Regiae (*Hu Tao Guo Pi*), 1500g, toad skin (*Ha Ma Pi*), 10 pieces, Borneol (*Bing Pian*), 9g

Method of preparation: Boil the above medicinals, except the Borneol, in a pot for 3 hours and then remove the dregs. Continue to reduce the concentrated juice with a mild fire down to 1000g. Then place it in a porcelain jar and add the powdered Borneol. Mix thoroughly and seal tightly for use.

Method of use: Apply to the affected area and change 1 time per day.

Functions: Resolves toxins, softens the hard, eliminates odor, and dispels necrosis

Indications: Bone toxins (*i.e.*, deeply rooted ulcerations affecting the bone) of all kinds and rupture of osteomyelitis which are productive of pus and serous fluid with an extremely repulsive odor

Commentary: This is an effective prescription often used by Monk Zhen Jun in the treatment of osteomyelitis.

106. *Shao Lin San Huang Gao*
Shaolin Three Yellows Plaster

Ingredients: Realgar (*Xiong Huang*), 12g, Sulfur 12g (*Liu Huang*), Radix Et Rhizoma Rhei (*Da Huang*), 30g, Secretio Bufonis (*Chan Su*), 1g, Borneol (*Bing Pian*), 3g, raw Radix Glycyrrhizae (*Sheng Gan Cao*), 21g

Method of preparation: Grind the Rhubarb root and the raw Licorice into a fine powder and sieve. Then grind the Realgar and mix it with the rest of the medicinals. Keep in air-tight bottles for use.

Method of use: When needed, take some of this powder and mix it with aged vinegar and make into a paste. Apply it to the affected area and change the dressing 1 time per day.

Functions: Resolves toxins, stops itching, and eliminates necrosis

Indications: Ulcerous conditions due to metal weapons, intolerable itching of a deeply rooted ulcer, pernicious, necrotic wounds producing toxic pus, unaccountable toxic swellings, and insect bites

107. *Shao Lin Jie Du Gao*
Shaolin Toxin-resolving Plaster

Ingredients: Blackened toad (*Hei Ha Ma*), 9g, Sulfur (*Liu Huang*), 12g, Realgar (*Xiong Huang*), 9g, Borneol (*Bing Pian*), 3g, highest quality white alcohol (*Bai Jiu*)

Method of preparation: Grind the above 4 medicinals into a fine powder and mix into a dilute paste with some fine white alcohol. Keep this in a tightly closed porcelain jar for use.

Method of use: Apply to the affected area.

Functions: Resolves toxins, kills parasites, stops itching, and stops pain

Indications: Insect bites of all kinds, localized redness, swelling, and pain, and burning and itching sensations

Commentary: This prescription has been passed down from a monk called Yong Xiang. It is especially effective for treating the bites of scorpions, centipedes, and poisonous spiders.

108. *Shao Lin Wan Ying Gao*
Shaolin Ten Thousand Respondings Plaster

Ingredients: Radix Angelicae Sinensis (*Dang Gui*), 30g, Radix Angelicae (*Bai Zhi*), 30g, Gummum Olibani (*Ru Xiang*, vinegar processed), 15g, Myrrha (*Mo Yao*, vinegar processed), 15g, Flos Lonicerae Japonicae (*Jin Yin Hua*), 30g, Radix Rubrus Paeoniae Lactiflorae (*Chi Shao*), 30g, Acacia Catechu (*Er Cha*), 15g, Flos Carthami Tinctorii (*Hong Hua*), 30g, Radix Ledebouriellae Sesloidis (*Fang Feng*), 15g, Flos Seu Herba Schizonepetae Tenuifoliae (*Jing Jie Sui*), 15g, Os Tigridis (*Hu Gu*), 9g, Buthus Martensi (*Quan Chong*), 9g, Rhizoma Gastrodiae Elatae (*Tian Ma0*, 9g, Fructus Chaenomelis Lagenariae (*Mu Gua*), 30g, Lignum Sappanis (*Su Mu*), 9g, Herba Artimisiae Anomalae (*Liu Ji Nu*), 9g, Sanguis Draconis (*Xue Jie*), 6g, Squama Manitis Pentadactylis (*Chuan Shan Jia*), 12g, Lignum Santali Albi (*Bai Tan Xiang*), 12g, Eupolyphaga Seu Opisthoplatia (*Tu Bie Chong*), 6g, Semen Strychnotis (*Ma Qian Zi*), 12g, Ramulus Cinnamomi (*Gui Zhi*), 12g, Rhizoma Homalomenae (*Qian Nian Jian*), 9g, Radix Cyathulae (*Chuan Niu Xi*), 30g, Caulis Millettiae Seu Spatholobi (*Ji Xue Teng*), 30g, Ramulus Mori Albi (*Sang Zhi*), 30g, Pyritum (*Zi Ran Tong*), 6g, Radix Stephaniae Tetrandrae (*Han Fan Ji*), 18g, Caulis Photiniae Serrulatae (*Shi Nan*

Teng), 18g, Caulis Sinomenii (*Qing Feng Teng*), 18g, Radix Aconiti (*Chuan Wu*), 12g, Radix Aconiti (*Cao Wu*), 12g, Radix Dipsaci (*Chuan Duan*), 30g, Radix Saussureae Seu Vladimiriae (*Mu Xiang*), 12g, Rhizoma Corydalis Yanhusuo (*Yan Hu Suo*), 30g, Rhizoma Atractylodis (*Cang Zhu*), 12g, Radix Gentianae Macrophyllae (*Qin Jiao*), 30g, Semen Cnidii Monnieri (*She Chuang Zi*), 12g, Cortex Radicis Dictamni Dasycarpi (*Bai Xian Pi*), 15g, Radix Sophorae Flavescentis (*Ku Shen*), 12g, Herba Erodii Seu Geranii (*Nian Guan Cao*), 15g, Fructus Xanthii (*Cang Er Zi*), 15g, Agkistrodon Seu Bungarus (*Bai Hua She*), 30g, Radix Trichosanthis Kirlowii (*Tian Hua Fen*), 30g, Herba Cum Radice Violae Yedoensis (*Di Ding*), 15g, Herba Cum Radice Taraxaci Mongolici (*Pu Gong Ying*), 30g, Radix Et Rhizoma Rhei (*Da Huang*), 30g, Sichuan Rhizoma Coptidis Chinensis (*Chuan Huang Lian*), 30g, Cortex Phellodendri (*Huang Bai*), 15g, Semen Pruni Persicae (*Tao Ren*), 15g, Rhizoma Sparganii (*San Leng*), 15g, Rhizoma Curcumae Zedoariae (*E Zhu*), 15g, Realgar (*Xiong Huang*), 13g, Alum (*Bai Fan*), 15g, Secretio Moschi Moschiferi (*She Xiang*), 6g, Borneol (*Bing Pian*), 9g, Minium (*Guang Dan*), 600g, roasted sesame oil (*Xiang You*), 3kg

Method of preparation: Among the above 57 ingredients, grind the Musk, Realgar, Alum, Sanguis Draconis, Borneol, Pyritum, Acacia Catechu, Frankincense, and Myrrh into a fine powder separately. Then stir-fry the remaining 48 ingredients in a pot filled with the oil until the medicinals have been burnt. Filter and continue to heat the oil. When ripples appear on the surface of the oil moving out from the center to the sides of the pot, take the pot off the fire and add the Minium (all the while stirring the oil to prevent lumping and burning). The ratio between the medicated oil and the Minium should be 300g to 90g.

Pour the oil into cold water in which the oil should be left immersed for 15 days. Change the water 2 times per day so as to clear the fire toxins. Cut the paste into small pieces and rinse with water before steaming. Lastly, add the 8 powdered ingredients and mix them thoroughly into the plaster.

Spreading the plasters: a plaster 8cm long should weigh 9g, whereas one 5cm long should weigh 6g and one 3cm should weigh 3g.

Functions: Quickens the blood and dispels stasis, disperse swelling and stops pain, soothes the sinews and quickens the joints, expels wind and scatters cold, settles tetany, kills worms, and stops itching, breaks accumulations and disperses gatherings, reunites the sinews and connects the bones.

It is indicated for the treatment of swelling and pain due to blood stasis, low back strain, and *shan* pain of the lumbar region and thighs, numbness of the four limbs, inhibition of the joints, spastic limbs, hemiplegia, wind, damp, and cold *bi*, difficulty in walking, twitching and tremor, deviation of the mouth and eyes, fractures and dislocations, wind evils skin itching, concretions and conglomerations in the abdomen, and hard to bear pain due to blood accumulation and qi accumulation

Method of use: The effect of this treatment will be improved if the affected area is also treated with *tui na* (*i.e.*, Chinese remedial massage), *an mo* (*i.e.*, Chinese folk massage), or *zhen jiu* (*i.e.*, acupuncture/moxibustion) before applying the plaster. A brief illustration of some common acupoints for clinical reference is as follows:

1. Chest pain: *Shan Zhong* (CV 17) & *Yu Tang* (CV 18)
2. Lateral costal pain: *Da Bao* (Sp 21)
3. Side of the chest pain: *Ying Chuang* (St 16) & *Ling Xu* (Ki 24)
4. Upper abdominal accumulation and lump: *Zhong Wan* (CV 12) & *Ju Que* (CV 14)

5. Lower abdominal accumulation and lump: *Qi Hai* (CV 6), *Zhong Ji* (CV 3) & *Tian Shu* (St 25)
6. Low back pain: *Shen Shu* (Bl 23), *Ming Men* (GV 4) & *Wei Zhong* (Bl 40)
7. Lumbosacral pain: *Shang Liao* (Bl 31) & *Xia Liao* (Bl 34)
8. Hip pain: *Huan Tiao* (GB 30) & *Feng Shi* (GB 31)
9. Numbness & paralysis of the lower limbs: *Yang Ling Quan* (GB 34), *Cheng Shan* (Bl 57) & *Kun Lun* (Bl 60)
10. Numbness & paralysis of the upper limbs: *Jian Yu* (LI 15), *Qu Chi* (LI 11) & *He Gu* (LI 4)
11. Injury of the wrist: *Nei Guan* (Per 6)
12. Injury of the dorsum of the foot: *Rang Gu* (Ki 2) & *Chong Yang* (St 42)
13. Injury of the ankle: *Jie Xi* (St 41) & *Shang Qiu* (Sp 5)
14. Injury of the upper arm: *Tian Fu* (Lu 3), *Bi Nao* (LI 14) & *Jian Yu* (LI 15)

In case of localized injury due to fall and strike, the plaster can be used after treating with massage. Change the plaster every 7 days.

Commentary: This is a secret prescription favored by the monk Xiao Shan, a Shaolin martial arts instructor during the Ming Dynasty. Eight to 900 cases of the above problems have been treated by De Chan, the contemporary Patriarch and monk doctor, with this formula proving its efficacy.

109. *Shao Lin Tang Shang Gao*
Shaolin Scalding Injury Plaster

Ingredients: Cortex Phellodendri (*Huang Bai*), 30g, Radix Et Rhizoma Rhei (*Da Huang*), 30g, Rhizoma Coptidis Chinensis (*Huang Lian*), 30g, Cortex Radicis Moutan (*Dan Pi*), 30g, Radix Scutellariae Baicalensis (*Huang Qin*), 30g, raw Radix Sanguisorbae (*Sheng Di Yu*), 90g, egg yolk (*Ji Huang You*), 30g, Borneol (*Bing Pian*), 6g

Method of preparation: Grind the first 6 ingredients into a fine powder and sieve. Then grind the Borneol and add it to the other powdered medicinals. Mix these together thoroughly and then make into a paste with the egg yolks. Raw sesame oil (*Sheng Xiang You*) can be added if more fluid is needed. Fill the paste in bottles and store with air-tight lids.

Method of use: Clean the affected area first before applying the plaster, which should be covered with white gauze (except in summer). Change the dressing every day. Three to 5 treatments will cure the patient. For critical scalding cases, approximately 15-20 treatments will be necessary before recovery.

110.   *Shao Lin Ban Jun Gao*
Shaolin Gentleman's Companion Plaster

Ingredients: Human cranium (*Tian Ling Kai*), 30g, Radix Angelicae (*Bai Zhi*), 60g, Sichuan Rhizoma Coptidis Chinensis (*Chuan Huang Lian*), 60g, Ramulus Cinnamomi (*Gui Zhi*), 30g, Camphora (*Chao Nao*), Menthol (*Bo He Bing*) 15g each, Borneol (*Bing Pian*), 6g, Secretio Moschi Moschiferi (*She Xiang*), 0.6g

Grind into a fine powder and make into a paste with raw sesame oil (*Sheng Xiang You*). Store in an air-tight container for use.

Method of use: For forehead pain, apply the plaster to *Yin Tang*. For migrainous pain, apply the plaster to *Tai Yang*. For pain at the vertex, apply to *Bai Hui* (GV 20). For dizziness and vertigo, apply to *Shang Xing* (GV 23) and *Feng Chi* (GB 20).

Functions: Rouses the spirit, clears the brain, opens the portals, and stops pain

Indications: Headache, blurred vision, listlessness, vertigo due to summerheat stroke

Commentary: As an effective ready-made medicament, this plaster is suitable for travel and sight-seeing for the prevention of injury due to summerheat and wind.

Chapter Six

Shaolin Folk & Home Remedies

111. *Gan Yan Si Zhi Xue Fang*
Dryland Pipe Tobacco Stop Bleeding Rx

For all types of bleeding due to external injury, take good quality tobacco leaves which have been baked brown and crush them by rolling. Spread these over the wound and press tightly. This will instantly stop the bleeding.

112. *Nei Wai Shang Zhi Xue Fang*
Rx to Stop Bleeding from Internal or External Injury

For the treatment of hemorrhage due either to external injury or injury to the internal viscera and bowels, fresh Herba Verbenae (*Xian Ma Deng Cao*) is preferred for its specific effect. In case of external injury, some fresh Herba Verbenae should be crushed and then pressed to the wound in order to stop the bleeding. In case of hemorrhage due to internal injury, take 30g of Herba Verbenae, decoct, and take internally. This will also check internal bleeding.

113. *Zhi Shang Hou Liang Bian Chu Xue Fang*
Rx for the Treatment of Post-injury Hemafecia & Hematuria

Radix Pseudoginseng (*San Qi*), 30g, Rhizoma Corydalis Yanhusuo (*Yan Hu Suo*), 15g, carbonized Fructus Crataegi (*Shan Zha Tan*), 30g, Herba Verbenae (*Ma Deng Cao*), 9g, carbonized Pollen Typhae (*Pu Huang Tan*), 24g

Grind these into fine powder. Take 9-15g each time, 3 times per day.

Commentary: Patriarch Zhen Zhu once cured over 50 cases with this prescription. Hence the name *Yu Gong San* (Abundant Public Affairs Powder) which is believed to have been given by the great monk Fu Hu of Shaolin Monastery in the Song Dynasty.

Chapter Seven

Formulas for the Treatment of Injury Due to *Dian Xue* or Spotting[1]

114. Rx for the Treatment of Spotting Injury to *Tan Men* (*i.e., Qi Men*, Liv 14)[2]

For lockjaw and a mouth that will not open, eyes staring upward, loss of consciousness due to blood inversion, first take *Duo Ming Dan* (Extend Life Elixir). If the upper part is also injured, take *Zi Jin Dan* (Purple Gold Elixir) in order to dispel blood stasis. After that, take Flos Carthami Tinctorii (*Hong Hua*), 12g, Semen Pruni Persicae (*Tao*

---

[1] Spotting is an advanced *wu shu* fighting technique where one attacks acupoints on their opponent, usually with internal power and often at specific times computed by calculating the stems and branches similar to computing acupuncture open points. Often, problems develop only days after the original attack as the qi reaches its target internally according to the rules and rhythms of its circulation.

[2] Many acupoints have more than one name as evidenced by the numerous alternatives listed in the *Zhen Jiu Da Cheng, (Great Compendium of Acupuncture and Moxibustion)*. Many of the points discussed in this chapter are identified by their traditional Shaolin names. Their standard TCM identifications are given in parentheses accompanied by their standard Western numerical notation.

Ren), 6g, Radix Rubrus Paeoniae Lactiflorae (*Chi Shao*), 12g, Fructus Citri Seu Ponciri (*Zhi Qiao*), 6g. Two *ji* should be effective.

115. Rx ... *Xue Qi (i.e., Yang Ling Quan,* GB 34)

Os Tigridis (*Hu Gu*), 6g, Radix Dipsaci (*Chuan Duan*), 6g, Radix Achyranthis Bidentatae (*Niu Xi*), 6g, Fructus Chaenomelis Lagenariae (*Mu Gua*), 6g, Radix Angelicae Sinensis tails (*Gui Wei*), 4.5g, Ramulus Cinnamomi (*Gui Zhi*), 3g, Rhizoma Drynariae (*Gu Sui Bu*), 6g, Cortex Eucommiae Ulmoidis (*Du Zhong*), 6g

Decoct the above medicinals with infant's urine and take internally. Take 1 time per day. The patient will be cured after 3 days' dosage.

116. Rx ... *Xue Chi (i.e., Xue Hai,* Sp 10)

Radix Achyranthis Bidentatae (*Niu Xi*), 4.5g, Radix Angelicae Sinensis (*Dang Gui*), 4.5g, Cortex Cinnamomi (*Rou Gui*), 4.5g, Rhizoma Ligustici Wallichii (*Chuan Xiong*), 4.5g, Flos Lonicerae Japonicae (*Jin Yin Hua*), 3g, Pericarpium Citri Reticulatae (*Chen Pi*), 3g, Herba Dendrobii (*Shi Hu*), 3g, Rhizoma Drynariae (*Gu Sui Bu*), 4.5g, Os Tigridis (*Hu Gu*), 4.5g, Radix Dipsaci (*Chuan Duan*), 4.5g

Mix the above medicinals with equal parts water and wine and decoct into a very thick juice. Ten *ji* equal 1 course of treatment.

117. Rx ... *Qi Kou (Bai Lao,* EX-HN15)

Cortex Cinnamomi (*Rou Gui*), 3g, Massa Medica Fermentata (*Shen Qu*), 6g, Radix Angelicae Sinensis (*Dang Gui*), 6g, Flos Carthami Tinctorii (*Hong Hua*), 9g, Tuber Ophiopogonis Japonicae (*Cun Dong*), 3g, Fructus Citri Seu Ponciri (*Zhi Qiao*), 3g, Pericarpium Citri Reticulatae (*Chen Pi*), 9g, Os Draconis (*Long Gu*), 9g, Lignum Aquilariae Agallochae (*Chen Xiang*), 1.5g, Rhizoma Sparganii (*San*

Formulas for the Treatment of Injury Due to *Dian Xue* or Spotting

Leng), 4.5g, Rhizoma Curcumae Zedoariae (*E Zhu*), 6g, raw Rhizoma Zingiberis (*Sheng Jiang*), 3 slices, raw Radix Glycyrrhizae (*Sheng Gan Cao*), 6g

Mix above medicinals in equal parts water and wine), decoct, and take.

118. Rx ... *Shen Guan (i.e., Shen Men*, Ht 7)

Radix Rehmanniae (*Sheng Di*), 9g, Radix Pseudoginseng (*San Qi*, take separately), 3g, Sanguis Draconis (*Xue Jie*), 3g, Sclerotium Poriae Cocos (*Fu Ling*), 9g, Radix Rubrus Paeoniae Lactiflorae (*Chi Shao*), 9g, Radix Angelicae Sinensis (*Dang Gui*), 6g, Pericarpium Citri Reticulatae (*Chen Pi*), 6g, Radix Glycyrrhizae (*Gan Cao*), 1.5g, Herba Allii Fistulosi (*Cong Bai*), 3 stalks

Add above medicinals to equal parts water and wine, decoct, and take.

119. Rx ... *Ming Gong (i.e., Ming Men*, GV 4)

Radix Glehniae Littoralis (*Sha Shen*), 9g, Radix Angelicae Sinensis (*Dang Gui*), 6g, Flos Carthami Tinctorii (*Hong Hua*), 3g, Fructus Citri Seu Ponciri (*Zhi Qiao*), 3g, Semen Cuscutae (*Tu Si Zi*), 9g, Cortex Magnoliae Officinalis (*Hou Po*), 3g, Sanguis Draconis (*Xue Jie*), 6g, Herba Cum Radice Asari (*Xi Xin*), 1.5g, Tuber Ophiopogonis Japonicae (*Cun Dong*), 6g, Feces Trogopterori Seu Pteromi (*Wu Ling Zhi*), 9g, Pyritum (*Zi Ran Tong*), 6g, raw Rhizoma Zingiberis (*Sheng Jiang*), 3 slices

Decoct with water, add 1 cup infant's urine, and take internally.

Secret Shaolin Formulas

120. Rx ... *Qiao Bun* (i.e., *Zhu Bin*, Ki 9)

Radix Angelicae Sinensis (*Dang Gui*), 6g, Rhizoma Ligustici Wallichii (*Chuan Xiong*), 9g, Radix Albus Paeoniae Lactiflorae (*Bai Shao*), 4.5g, Rhizoma Gastrodiae Elatae (*Tian Ma*), 1.5g, Radix Angelicae (*Bai Zhi*), 3g, Cortex Cinnamomi (*Rou Gui*), 3g, Radix Pseudoginseng (*San Qi*, pulverize & take separately), 6g, Radix Glycyrrhizae (*Gan Cao*), 6g, Radix Aristolochiae Seu Cocculi (*Xin Gu Feng*), 6g

Grind the above 9 medicinals into a fine powder and mix with yellow wine (*i.e.*, rice wine). Take 3-6g per dose, 2 times per day.

121. Rx ... *Wai Shen* (i.e., *Gao Wan*, testes)

An assistant should stand behind the back of the patient. The doctor should use both hands to press both sides of the lower abdomen downward. If this does not work, (*i.e.*, if the testicles do not descend), bathe the entire body in a decoction of 30g each of *Xi Zi Cai* (喜子菜) and salted pickled cabbage (*Xian Suan Cai*).

122. Rx ... *Wei Gong*

Semen Plantaginis (*Che Qian Zi*), 4.5g. Powder and take with rice soup. Or take Herba Ephedrae (*Ma Huang*), 3g, Radix Ledebouriellae Sesloidis (*Fang Feng*), 9g, Flos Carthami Tinctorii (*Hong Hua*), 4.5g, Semen Pruni Persicae (*Tao Ren*), 9g, Radix Rubrus Paeoniae Lactiflorae (*Chi Shao*), 9g, raw Radix Glycyrrhizae (*Sheng Gan Cao*), 6g

Decoct with water and take for good results.

Note: This point is located halfway between *Hui Yin* (CV 1) and the anus.

Formulas for the Treatment of Injury Due to *Dian Xue* or Spotting

123. Rx ... *Xiao Du Pang* (*i.e., Da Heng*, Sp 15)

First take *Zi Jin Dan* (Purple Gold Elixir; for ingredients see Appendix). Follow this by a decoction of Herba Artimisiae Capillaris (*Yin Chen Hao*).

124. Rx ... *Feng Guan* (*i.e., Feng Chi*, GB 20)

Eggplant skin (*Qie Pi*), 6g, Flos Carthami Tinctorii (*Hong Hua*), 3g, Radix Saussureae Seu Vladimiriae (*Mu Xiang*), 3g, Radix Glycyrrhizae (*Gan Cao*), 1.5g, Ramus Loranthi Seu Visci (*Sang Ji Sheng*), 9g, dry Radix Puerariae Lobatae (*Ge Gen*), 4.5g, Os Tigridis (*Hu Gu*), 9g, Cortex Cinnamomi (*Rou Gui*), 3g, Caulis Akebiae Mutong (*Mu Tong*), 3g, processed Rhizoma Pinelliae Ternatae (*Ban Xia*), 4.5g, Eupolyphaga Seu Opisthoplatia (*Tu Bie Chong*), 9g, Squama Manitis Pentadactylis (*Chuan Shan Jia*), 9g, processed Gummum Olibani (*Ru Xiang*), 9g, processed Myrrha (*Mo Yao*), 9g, Fructus Psoraleae Corylifoliae (*Bu Gu Zhi*), 9g, Herba Allii Fistulosi (*Cong Bai*), 3 stalks

Add the above medicinals to equal parts water and wine, decoct, and take.

125. Rx ... *Shen Shu* (Bl 23)

Radix Rehmanniae (*Sheng Di*), 9g, Radix Lindera Strychnifoliae (*Wu Yao*), 6g, Lignum Sappanis (*Su Mu*), 9g, Radix Lithospermi Seu Arnebiae (*Zi Cao*), 9g, processed Gummum Olibani (*Ru Xiang*), 9g, Fructus Chaenomelis Lagenariae (*Mu Gua*), 3g, Cortex Eucommiae Ulmoidis (*Du Zhong*), 9g, Radix Glycyrrhizae (*Gan Cao*), 1.5g

Decoct with water and take. One *ji* per day. If infant's urine is added, the effect will be better.

126. Rx ... *Feng Wei*

Radix Et Rhizoma Notopterygii (*Qiang Huo*), 3g, Radix Linderae Strychnifoliae (*Wu Yao*), 3g, processed Rhizoma Pinelliae Ternatae (*Ban Xia*), 4.5g, Flos Carthami Tinctorii (*Hong Hua*), 3g, Stalactitum (*Chong Ru Shi*), 9g, Sanguis Draconis (*Xue Jie*), 3g, Semen Arecae Catechu (*Bing Lang*), 4.5g, Radix Saussureae Seu Vladimiriae (*Mu Xiang*), 3g, Fructus Foeniculi Vulgaris (*Xiao Hui Xiang*), 3g, Fructus Psoraleae Corylifoliae (*Bu Gu Zhi*), 9g, Cortex Radicis Moutan (*Dan Pi*), 1.5g, Caulis Akebiae Mutong (*Mu Tong*), 3g, Semen Pruni Persicae (*Tao Ren*), 9g, Fructus Piperis Negri (*Hu Jiao*), 3g, raw Rhizoma Zingiberis (*Sheng Jiang*), 2 slices

To the above medicinals, add equal parts water and wine and decoct. Then add 1 cup infant's urine. Take the entire decoction in 1 dose.

Note: *Feng Wei* is located 8 *fen* lateral to *Ming Men*.

127. Rx ... *Tian Ping* (i.e., *Shen Ting*, GV 24)

Sanguis Draconis (*Xue Jie*), 6g, Os Tigridis (*Hu Gu*), 6g, Radix Pseudoginseng (*San Qi*, powder & take separately), 3g, Radix Glycyrrhizae (*Gan Cao*), 1.5g, precipitate of human urine (*Ren Zhong Bai*), 3g, goat's blood (*Shan Yang Xue*), 3g, Pyritum (*Zi Ran Tong*, dipped in vinegar 7 times), 6g, Terra Flava Usta (*Fu Long Gan*), 12g

Decoct above medicinals in water and take.

128. Rx ... *Feng Men* (Bl 12)

Radix Platycodi Grandiflori (*Jie Geng*), 3g, Cortex Radicis Moutan (*Dan Pi*), 4.5g, Flos Carthami Tinctorii (*Hong Hua*), 3g, Caulis Akebiae Mutong (*Mu Tong*), 3g, Fructus Psoraleae Corylifoliae (*Bu Gu Zhi*), 9g, Fructus Chaenomelis Lagenariae (*Mu Gua*), 3g, Radix

Pseudoginseng (*San Qi*, powder and take separately), 6g, Fructus Illici Veri (*Da Hui Xiang*), 3g, Radix Angelicae Pubescentis (*Du Huo*), 3g, Cortex Cinnamomi (*Rou Gui*), 3g, Radix Glycyrrhizae (*Gan Cao*), 1.5g, Gummum Olibani (*Ru Xiang*, remove the oil), 4.5g, Myrrha (*Mo Yao*, remove the oil), 4.5g, Sclerotium Poriae Cocos (*Fu Ling*), 9g, Terra Flava Usta (*Fu Long Gan*), 30g

Cook all the above medicinals in equal parts wine and water and take.

If the patient still does not recover, an alternative prescription consists of Talcum (*Hua Shi*), 12g, Cinnabar (*Zhu Sha*, grind in water & take separately), 3g, Os Draconis (*Long Gu*), 9g, Radix Linderae Strychnifoliae (*Wu Yao*), 3g, precipitate of human urine (*Ren Zhong Bai*), 6g, Sclerotium Pararadix Poriae Cocos (*Fu Shen*), 9g, Radix Gentianae Macrophyllae (*Qin Jiao*), 4.5g, Radix Glycyrrhizae (*Gan Cao*), 1.5g, Radix Dipsaci (*Chuan Duan*), 6g, Cortex Cercis Chinensis (*Zi Jing Pi*), 4.5g, Fructus Zizyphi Jujubae (*Hong Zao*), 3 pieces, roasted Semen Nelumbinis Nuciferae (*Lian Zi*), 7 kernels, Cortex Magnoliae Officinalis (*Hou Po*), 3g.

Decoct in water and take.

129. Rx ... *Bai Hui* (GV 20)

Rhizoma Ligustici Wallichii (*Chuan Xiong*), 6g, Radix Angelicae Sinensis (*Dang Gui*), 6g, Radix Rubrus Paeoniae Lactiflorae (*Chi Shao*), 3g, Rhizoma Cimicifugae (*Sheng Ma*), 2.4g, Radix Ledebouriellae Sesloidis (*Fang Feng*), 2.4g, Flos Carthami Tinctorii (*Hong Hua*), 1.2g, Gummum Olibani (*Ru Xiang*, remove the oil), 1.2g, Pericarpium Citri Reticulatae (*Chen Pi*), 1.5g, Radix Glycyrrhizae (*Gan Cao*), 0.6g

Decoct with water and take.

130. Rx ... *Tai Yang* (EX-HN5)

Radix Angelicae Sinensis (*Dang Gui*), 6g, Flos Carthami Tinctorii (*Hong Hua*), 4.5g, Radix Astragali Membranacei (*Huang Qi*), 4.5g, Radix Angelicae (*Bai Zhi*), 4.5g, Rhizoma Cimicifugae (*Sheng Ma*), 4.5g, Pericarpium Citri Reticulatae (*Chen Pi*), 4.5g, Herba Seu Flos Schizonepetae Tenuifoliae (*Jing Jie Sui*), 5.4g, Cortex Cinnamomi (*Rou Gui*), 3g, Rhizoma Ligustici Wallichii (*Chuan Xiong*), 5.4g, Radix Glycyrrhizae (*Gan Cao*), 3.6g

Decoct with water and then add 1 cup of infant's urine and 1.5g yellow wine (*i.e.*, rice wine). Take internally.

131. Rx ... *Hong Tang*

Radix Et Rhizoma Rhei (*Da Huang*), 2.4g, carbonized septum of hairy bamboo (*Mao Zhu Jie*), 1.5g, pine cones (*Song Tou*, carbonized), 1.5g

Grind the medicinals into powder. Each dose is 1.5-3g. Take with yellow wine (*i.e.*, rice wine).

Note: *Hong Tang* is located 2 *fen* above *Yin Tang* (M-HN-3).

132. Rx ... *Zhi Shi* (Bl 52)

Radix Clematidis Chinensis (*Wei Ling Xian*), 3g, Ramulus Cinnamomi (*Gui Zhi*), 3g, Rhizoma Ligustici Wallichii (*Chuan Xiong*), 3g, Radix Dipsaci (*Chuan Duan*), 3g, Semen Pruni Persicae (*Tao Ren*), 3g, Pericarpium Citri Reticulatae (*Chen Pi*), 2.4g, Radix Glycyrrhizae (*Gan Cao*), 0.9g, Radix Angelicae Sinensis (*Dang Gui*), 4.5g

Formulas for the Treatment of Injury Due to *Dian Xue* or Spotting

Decoct in water, add 30g of yellow wine (*i.e.*, rice wine), mix well, and take internally.

133.   Rx ... *Jian Wo (i.e., Jian Yu,* LI 15)

Lignum Sappanis (*Su Mu*), 4.5g, Fructus Chaenomelis Lagenariae (*Mu Gua*, carbonized), 4.5g, carbonized septum of hairy bamboo (*Mao Zhu Jie*), 4.5g, Radix Angelicae Sinensis tails (*Gui Wei*), 3g, Rhizoma Cimicifugae (*Sheng Ma*), 4.5g, Rhizoma Ligustici Wallichii (*Chuan Xiong*), 3g

Powder the above medicinals and take with yellow wine (*i.e.*, rice wine), 1-3g per dose.

134.   Rx ... *Ming Mai (i.e., Tai Yuan,* Lu 9)

Radix Angelicae Sinensis tails (*Gui Wei*), 9g, Radix Lithospermi Seu Arnebiae (*Zi Cao*), 4.5g, Lignum Sappanis (*Su Mu*), 4.5g, Flos Carthami Tinctorii (*Hong Hua*), 4.5g, Cortex Cinnamomi (*Rou Gui*), 3g, Pericarpium Citri Reticulatae (*Chen Pi*), 3g, Fructus Citri Seu Ponciri (*Zhi Qiao*), 3g, Herba Dendrobii (*Shi Hu*), 1.5g, Radix Glycyrrhizae (*Gan Cao*), 1.5g

Place the above medicinals in equal amounts of water and wine and decoct. Add 1 cup infant's urine and take internally for good effect.

135.   Rx ... *Mai Zong (i.e., Nei Guan,* Per 6)

Radix Angelicae Sinensis tails (*Gui Wei*), 3g, Radix Dipsaci (*Chuan Duan*), 3g, Semen Pruni Persicae (*Tao Ren*), 3g, Fructus Citri Seu Ponciri (*Zhi Qiao*), 4.5g, Herba Artimisiae Anomalae (*Liu Ji Nu*), 3g, Flos Carthami Tinctorii (*Hong Hua*), 3g, Radix Glycyrrhizae (*Gan Cao*), 0.6g, Nodus Nelumbinis Nuciferae (*Ou Jie*), 9g, Rhizoma

Drynariae (*Gu Sui Bu*), 9g, goat's blood (*Shan Yang Xue*, take separately), 0.9g

Decoct with water and take. Each day 1 *ji* for 3 days.

136. Rx ... *Tan Tu*[3]

Radix Angelicae Sinensis (*Dang Gui*), 3g, Rhizoma Ligustici Wallichii (*Chuan Xiong*), 3g, Flos Carthami Tinctorii (*Hong Hua*), 3g, Pericarpium Arecae Catechu (*Da Fu Pi*), 3g, Rhizoma Drynariae (*Gu Sui Bu*), 3g, Herba Seu Flos Schizonepetae Tenuifoliae (*Jing Jie Sui*), 2.4g, Semen Pruni Armeniacae (*Xing Ren*), 2.4g, Radix Lithospermi Seu Arnebiae (*Zi Cao*), 2.4g, Folium Perillae Frutescentis (*Zi Su Ye*), 2.4g, carbonized black Fructificatio Tremellae (*Hei Mu Er Tan*), 4.5g, Medulla Junci (*Deng Xin Cao*), 0.9g

Decoct the above medicinals in equal parts water and wine and take.

137. Rx ... *Xuan Ji* (i.e., *Xuan Ji*, CV 21)

Lake bamboo root (*Hu Zhu Gen*), golden pheasant tree root (*Jin Ji Shu Gen*), lion's head herb with root (*Shi Zi Tou Cao [Lian Gen]*), *Jin Qi Shu Gen* (槿漆树根, remove the heart), buckwheat root (*Tian Jie Mai Gen*, remove the skin), 1.5g each

To the above medicinals, add rice vinegar, decoct, and take. For hiccup and vomiting, add 1 spoon of fresh ginger juice (*Jiang Zhi*) and take warm.

Note: Abstain from fried foods and raw and cold foods.

---

[3] No location is given for this point in the text nor have we been able to identify it.

Formulas for the Treatment of Injury Due to *Dian Xue* or Spotting

138. Rx ... *Suo Xin (i.e., Jiu Wei*, CV 15)

Radix Et Rhizoma Rhei (*Da Huang*), 4.5g, hairy bamboo septa (*Mai Zhu Jie*, carbonized), 3g, Rhizoma Homalomenae (*Qian Nian Jian*, carbonized), 2.4g, pine cones (*Song Tou*, carbonized), 3g

Powder the above medicinals and take with yellow wine (*i.e.*, rice wine). Also take Semen Pruni Persicae (*Tao Ren*), 7 kernels, Flos Carthami Tinctorii (*Hong Hua*), 2.4g, Semen Sinapis Albae (*Bai Jie Zi*), 3g, Pericarpium Citri Reticulatae (*Chen Pi*), 5g, Fructus Citri Seu Ponciri (*Zhi Qiao*), 6g, Radix Et Rhizoma Notopterygii (*Qiang Huo*), 6g, Radix Angelicae Sinensis tails (*Gui Wei*), 6g, Cortex Cinnamomi (*Rou Gui*), 4.5g, Lignum Sappanis (*Su Mu*), 4.5g, Radix Rubrus Paeoniae Lactiflorae (*Chi Shao*), 1.5g, Radix Glycyrrhizae (*Gan Cao*), 0.6g, decocted with equal parts water and wine.

139. Rx ... *Fei Miao (i.e., Shu Fu*, Ki 27)

Radix Angelicae Sinensis tails (*Gui Wei*), 4.5g, Flos Carthami Tinctorii (*Hong Hua*), 2.4g, Pericarpium Citri Reticulatae (*Chen Pi*), 2.4g, Semen Pruni Armeniacae (*Xing Ren*), 2.4g, Semen Sinapis Albae (*Bai Jie Zi*), 3g, Myrrha (*Mo Yao*, remove the oil), 1.2g, Radix Angelicae Pubescentis (*Du Huo*), 1.5g, Herba Dendrobii (*Shi Hu*), 1.5g, Folium Perillae Frutescentis (*Zi Su Ye*), 1.5g, Radix Glycyrrhizae (*Gan Cao*), 1.5g

Decoct the above medicinals in equal parts water and wine and take.

140. Rx ... *Wan Xin (i.e., Da Ling*, Per 7)

Radix Angelicae Sinensis tails (*Gui Wei*), 3g, Pericarpium Citri Reticulatae (*Chen Pi*), 3g, Radix Dipsaci (*Chuan Duan*), 3g, Semen Sinapis Albae (*Bai Jie Zi*), 3g, Radix Et Rhizoma Rhei (*Da Huang*), 9g, Flos Carthami Tinctorii (*Hong Hua*), 1.5g, Radix Et Rhizoma

Notopterygii (*Qiang Huo*), 1.5g, Semen Pharbitidis (*Er Chou, i.e.*, black and white seeds), 4.5g, Radix Glycyrrhizae (*Gan Cao*), 1.2g, Folium Perillae Frutescentis (*Zi Su Ye*), 4.5g, Medulla Junci (*Deng Xin Cao*), 0.9g

Decoct in equal parts water and wine and take, 1 *ji* each day for 3 days.

141. Rx ... *Diao Jin*

Radix Clematidis Chinensis (*Wei Ling Xian*), 6g, Radix Dipsaci (*Chuan Duan*), 3g, Rhizoma Cibotti Barometsis (*Gou Ji*), 3g, Radix Angelicae Sinensis (*Dang Gui*), 3g, Os Tigridis (*Hu Gu*), 4.5g, Semen Pruni Persicae (*Tao Ren*), 0.6g, Herba Lophatheri Gracilis (*Dan Zhu Ye*), 1.2g, Folium Perillae Frutescentis (*Zi Su Ye*), 1.5g, Radix Ledebouriellae Sesloidis (*Fang Feng*), 1.5g, dry Rhizoma Zingiberis (*Gan Jiang*), 1.5g

Decoct the above medicinals in equal parts water and wine and take. Take 3 *ji*.

Note: *Diao Jin* is located 2 *fen* above *Zhang Men* (Liv 13).

142. Rx ... *Zhuan Xin* (i.e., *Xin Shu*, Bl 15)

Radix Et Rhizoma Rhei (*Da Huang*), 3g, Radix Angelicae Sinensis tails (*Gui Wei*), 3g, Rhizoma Ligustici Wallichii (*Chuan Xiong*), 2.4g, Radix Rubrus Paeoniae Lactiflorae (*Chi Shao*), 2.4g, Radix Et Rhizoma Notopterygii (*Qiang Huo*), 1.5g, Radix Bupleuri (*Chai Hu*), 1.5g, Flos Carthami Tinctorii (*Hong Hua*), 1.5g, Pericarpium Citri Reticulatae (*Chen Pi*), 1.8g, Radix Platycodi Grandiflori (*Jie Geng*), 1.8g, Radix Glycyrrhizae (*Gan Cao*), 0.6g

Formulas for the Treatment of Injury Due to *Dian Xue* or Spotting

Decoct the above 10 medicinal ingredients in equal parts water and wine and take.

143. Rx ... *Fei Shu* (Bl 13)

Semen Pruni Armeniacae (*Xing Ren*), 2.4g, Pericarpium Citri Reticulatae (*Chen Pi*), 2.4g, Lignum Dalbergiae Odoriferae (*Jiang Xiang*), 3g, Folium Perillae Frutescentis (*Zi Su Ye*), 3g, Radix Angelicae Sinensis (*Dang Gui*), 3g, Rhizoma Drynariae (*Gu Sui Bu*), 3g, Semen Sinapis Albae (*Bai Jie Zi*), 3g, Rhizoma Cimicifugae (*Sheng Ma*), 1.5g, Radix Glycyrrhizae (*Gan Cao*), 0.6g, Medulla Junci (*Deng Xin Cao*), 0.3g

Decoct the above medicinals in equal parts water and wine and take. If 1 cup of infant's urine is added, the results will be better.

144. Rx .. *Shi Cang* (i.e., *Xia Wan*, CV 10)

Goat's blood 0.9g (*Shan Yang Xue*, take separately), Radix Angelicae Sinensis (*Dang Gui*), 3g, Radix Lithospermi Seu Arnebiae (*Zi Cao*), 3g, Rhizoma Drynariae (*Gu Sui Bu*), 3g, Semen Sinapis Albae (*Bai Jie Zi*), 3g, Radix Et Rhizoma Rhei (*Da Huang*), 3g, Radix Et Rhizoma Notopterygii (*Qiang Huo*), 1.5g, Fructus Citri Seu Ponciri (*Zhi Qiao*), 1.5g, Herba Dendrobii (*Shi Hu*), 1.5g, Gummum Olibani (*Ru Xiang*, remove the oil), 2.4g, Radix Glycyrrhizae (*Gan Cao*), 0.6g, Medulla Junci (*Deng Xin Cao*), 0.3g

Decoct in equal parts water and wine and take.

145. Rx ... *Xue Chang* (i.e., *Ge Shu*, Bl 17)

Radix Angelicae Sinensis (*Dang Gui*), 3g, Radix Dipsaci (*Chuan Duan*), 3g, Herba Dendrobii (*Shi Hu*), 3g, Radix Rehmanniae (*Sheng Di*), 3g, Flos Carthami Tinctorii (*Hong Hua*), 1.5g, Pericarpium Citri

101

Reticulatae (*Chen Pi*), 1.5g, Radix Et Rhizoma Notopterygii (*Qiang Huo*), 1.5g, Radix Rubrus Paeoniae Lactiflorae (*Chi Shao*), 2.4g, Radix Glycyrrhizae (*Gan Cao*), 0.6g

Decoct in equal parts water and wine and add 1 cup infant's urine. Take internally.

146. Rx ... *Dan Zhu* (i.e., *Dan Shu*, Bl 19)

Radix Angelicae Sinensis (*Dang Gui*), 3g, Semen Pruni Persicae (*Tao Ren*), 10 kernels, Pericarpium Citri Reticulatae (*Chen Pi*), 1.5g, Radix Glycyrrhizae (*Gan Cao*), 1.5g, Medulla Junci Effusi (*Deng Xin Cao*), 0.3g

Decoct in equal parts water and wine and take.

147. Rx ... *You Guan* (i.e., *You Men*, Ki 21)

Cortex Cinnamomi (*Rou Gui*), 3g, Radix Angelicae Sinensis tails (*Gui Wei*), 3g, purple Flos Caryophylli (*Zi Ding Xiang*), 1.5g, Lignum Dalbergiae Odoriferae (*Jiang Xiang*), 1.5g, Pericarpium Citri Reticulatae (*Chen Pi*), 2.4g, Fructus Citri Seu Ponciri (*Zhi Qiao*), 2.4g, Fructus Perillae Frutescentis (*Zi Su Zi*), 4.5g, Radix Glycyrrhizae (*Gan Cao*), 0.6g

Decoct in equal parts water and yellow wine (*i.e.*, rice wine). Take 4 *ji*.

148. Rx ... *Tan Ning* (i.e., *Shan Zhong*, CV 17)

Folium Perillae Frutescentis (*Zi Su Ye*), 3g, Herba Seu Flos Schizonepetae Tenuifoliae (*jing Jie Sui*), 3g, Rhizoma Alpiniae Officinari (*Gao Liang Jiang*), 3g, Radix Et Rhizoma Notopterygii (*Qiang Huo*), 2.4g, Radix Angelicae Sinensis (*Dang Gui*), 2.4g, Semen Pruni Armeniacae (*Xing Ren*), 1.5g, Fructus Amomi (*Sha*

Formulas for the Treatment of Injury Due to *Dian Xue* or Spotting

Ren), 1.5g, Flos Carthami Tinctorii (*Hong Hua*), 1.5g, Fructus Citri Seu Ponciri (*Zhi Qiao*), 1.5g, Radix Glycyrrhizae (*Gan Cao*), 0.6g

Decoct in equal parts water and wine and take.

149. Rx ... Gan Jing[4]

Nodus Rhizomatis Nelumbinis Nuciferae (*Ou Jie*), 4.5g, Cortex Cinnamomi (*Rou Gui*), 3g, Radix Linderae Strychnifoliae (*Wu Yao*), 3g, Radix Dipsaci (*Chuan Duan*), 3g, Semen Sinapis Albae (*Bai Jie Zi*), 3g, Gummum Olibani (*Ru Xiang*, remove the oil), 3g, Radix Angelicae Sinensis (*Dang Gui*), 3g, Herba Artimisiae Anomalae (*Liu Ji Nu*), 2.4g, carbonized Fructificatio Tremellae (*Mu Er Tan*), 1.5g, Radix Glycyrrhizae (*Gan Cao*), 0.4g

Decoct in equal parts water and wine and take.

150. Rx ... Tian Zong (SI 11)

Iron rust (*Tie Xiu*), 1.2g, hairy bamboo septa (*Mao Zhu Jie*, carbonized), 1.5g, Rhizoma Homalomenae (*Qian Nian Jian*, carbonized), 1.5g, heartwood of Lignum Sappanis (*Su Mu Xin*), 1.5g, Lumbricus (*Di Long*), 4.5g

Powder the above medicinals and take with yellow wine (*i.e.*, rice wine).

---

[4] Point not identified.

151. Rx ... Shi Jie[5]

Radix Et Rhizoma Rhei (*Da Huang*), 9g, Fructus Germinatus Oryzae Sativae (*Gu Ya*), 9g, Rhizoma Curcumae Zedoariae (*E Zhu*), 3g, Rhizoma Ligustici Wallichii (*Chuan Xiong*), 3g, Pericarpium Citri Reticulatae (*Chen Pi*), 3g, Semen Pruni Persicae (*Tao Ren*), 3g, Fructus Crataegi (*Shan Zha*), 3g, Herba Dendrobii (*Shi Hu*), 3g, Radix Angelicae Sinensis (*Dang Gui*), 4.5g, Semen Sinapis Albae (*Bai Jie Zi*), 2.4g, Os Tigridis (*Hu Gu*), 3g, Radix Glycyrrhizae (*Gan Cao*), 0.6g

Decoct in yellow wine (*i.e.*, rice wine) and take.

152. Rx ... Hai Jiao

Rhizoma Ligustici Wallichii (*Chuan Xiong*), 3g, Pericarpium Citri Reticulatae (*Chen Pi*), 3g, Fructus Amomi (*Sha Ren*), 3g, Radix Angelicae (*Bai Zhi*), 4.5g, Radix Angelicae Sinensis (*Dang Gui*), 4.5g, Radix Et Rhizoma Rhei (*Da Huang*), 3g, Radix Glycyrrhizae (*Gan Cao*), 0.7g

Decoct the above medicinals in yellow wine (*i.e.*, rice wine), add infant's urine, and take 3 *ji*.

Note: Hai Jiao is located 3 *fen* lateral to *Qi Hai*.

153. Rx ... Qi Shi

Iron rust (*Tie Xiu*), 1.5g, Rhizoma Ligustici Wallichii (*Chuan Xiong*), 6g

---

[5] Point not identified.

Decoct the above 2 medicinals in water. If the patient has an external wound, *Bai Yu Gao* (White Jade Plaster) can be applied to the affected area.

Note: *Qi Shi* is located 2 *fen* below *Da Bao*.

154. Rx ... *Hua Gai*[6]

Rhizoma Ligustici Wallichii (*Chuan Xiong*), 6g, Radix Angelicae Sinensis tails (*Gui Wei*), 9g, Rhizoma Corydalis Yanhusuo (*Yan Hu Suo*), 6g, Radix Saussureae Seu Vladimiriae (*Mu Xiang*), 6g, Pericarpium Viridis Citri Reticulatae (*Qing Pi*), 6g, Radix Linderae Strychnifoliae (*Wu Yao*), 6g, Semen Pruni Persicae (*Tao Ren*), 6g, Radix Polygalae Tenuifoliae (*Yuan Zhi*), 6g, Rhizoma Sparganii (*San Leng*), 4.5g, Rhizoma Curcumae Zedoariae (*E Zhu*), 4.5g, Rhizoma Drynariae (*Gu Sui Bu*), 6g, Radix Rubrus Paeoniae Lactiflorae (*Chi Shao*), 6g, Lignum Sappanis (*Su Mu*), 6g, Fructus Citri Seu Ponciri (*Zhi Qiao*), 6g, Rhizoma Alpiniae Officinari (*Gao Liang Jiang*), 6g

Decoct with water and take internally.

Commentary: *Hua Gai* is a point on the lung channel. Injury to this point may cause death from coma due to overwhelming of the heart by blood. In acute cases, ingredients with an upbearing property are preferable. The purpose of these are to prevent stagnation and accumulation of the qi and blood. Upbearing ingredients should be added to 0.6g of *Shao Lin Qi Li San* (Shaolin 7 *Li* Powder) which should be taken with yellow wine (*i.e.*, rice wine). The effect of this treatment is to dispel stasis and quicken the blood, disperse swelling and stop pain. Also add 3-9g of *Shao Lin Duo Ming Dan* (Shaolin

---

[6] Point not identified.

Secret Shaolin Formulas

Extend the Life Elixir). Several days of treatment will bring back the patient.

155. Rx ... *Fei Du* (*i.e., Ri Yue*, GB 24)

If this point is injured, it may lead to death because of nasal hemorrhage in severe cases. To rescue the patient from such a critical condition, use Rx #192 below as the main prescription. To this add Cortex Radicis Mori Albi (*Sang Bai Pi*), 6g. Decoct in water. Take 0.4g of *Shao Lin Qi Li San* (Shaolin 7 *Li* Powder) and 3 *ji* of *Zi Jin Dan* (Purple Gold Elixir).

156. Rx ... *Zheng Qi*

Rx #192 plus Gummum Olibani (*Ru Xiang*, vinegar processed), 6g, Pericarpium Viridis Citri Reticulatae (*Qing Pi*), 6g. Decoct in water and take. Or one can take *Shao Lin Qi Li San* (Shaolin 7 *Li* Powder), 0.9g, and *Duo Ming Dan* (Extend the Life Elixir), 6g, 2 times per day. Take with yellow wine (*i.e.*, rice wine) for 3 days.

Note: *Zheng Qi* is located 2 *fen* above *Shan Zhong*.

157. Rx ... *Qi Hai* (CV 6)

Rx #192 plus Radix Saussureae Seu Vladimiriae (*Mu Xiang*), 6g, and Guangdong Pericarpium Citri Reticulatae (*Guang Chen Pi*), 6g. Decoct in water and take. If this is not effective, the above ingredients should be taken with *Qi Li San* (7 *Li* Powder) and *Duo Ming Dan* (Extend the Life Elixir).

158. Rx ... *Xue Hai* (Sp 10)

Rx #192 plus Radix Saussureae Seu Vladimiriae (*Mu Xiang*), 6g, Rhizoma Corydalis Yanhusuo (*Yan Hu Suo*), 6g. Decoct in water and

Formulas for the Treatment of Injury Due to *Dian Xue* or Spotting

take. Six tenths of a gram of *Qi Li San* (7 *Li* Powder) and 6g of *Duo Ming Dan* (Extend the Life Elixir) can be added in severe cases. Very effective!

159. Rx ... *Xia Xue Hai*[7]

Rx #192 plus Feces Trogopterori Seu Pteromi (*Wu Ling Zhi*), 4.5g, Pollen Typhae (*Pu Huang*), 4.5g. Decoct in water and take. Or one can take 0.7g of *Shao Lin Qi Li San* (Shaolin 7 *Li* Powder) and 3-6g of *Duo Ming Dan* (Extend the Life Elixir) with yellow wine (*i.e.*, rice wine).

160. Rx ... *Qi Xue Er Hai*[8]

Rx 1. Rx #192 plus Radix Saussureae Seu Vladimiriae (*Mu Xiang*) and Fructus Citri Seu Ponciri (*Zhi Qiao*), 4.5g each, decocted with water and taken.

Rx 2. Nine tenths of a gram of *Qi Li San* (7 *Li* Powder) and 3-6g of *Duo Ming Dan* (Extend the Life Elixir) taken with yellow wine (*i.e.*, rice wine).

Note: This point homes to the heart, liver, and lung channels. If it is injured, these three viscera will also be injured. If such injury is not cured within 7 days, it will be difficult to effect a cure afterward.

---

[7] Point not identified; however, judging from the name, this point seems to be just inferior to *Xue Hai* (Sp 10).

[8] Point not identified.

161. Rx ... Hei Fu (i.e., Shang Wan, CV 13)

Rx 1. Rx #192 plus Cortex Cinnamomi (*Rou Gui*), 3g, Purple Flos Caryophylli (*Zi Ding Xiang*), 1.8g. Decoct in water and take.

Rx 2. Nine tenths of a gram of *Qi Li San* (7 *Li* Powder) and 9g of *Duo Ming Dan* (Extend the Life Elixir) taken with yellow wine (*i.e.*, rice wine). Then take *Di Bie Zi Jin Dan* (Eupolyphaga Purple Gold Elixir), 3-6g.

Note: If this point is injured, the patient may become comatose immediately. If not cured within 12 days, recovery will be difficult.

162. Rx ... Huo Fei

Rx 1. Rx #192 plus Radix Platycodi Grandiflori (*Jie Geng*), 3g, Bulbus Fritillariae Cirrhosae (*Chuan Bei Mu*), 4.5g. Decoct with water and take.

Rx 2. Three to 6g of *Duo Ming Dan* (Extend the Life Elixir) and 0.7g of *Shao Lin Qi Li San* (Shaolin 7 *Li* Powder). Then take *Di Bie Zi Jin Dan* (Eupolyphaga Purple Gold Elixir[9]), 6g.

Note: This point homes to the heart channel. It is located 2 *fen* below *Fei Shu* (Bl 13). If it is injured, the patient will lose consciousness. If this condition is not cured in time, relapse may occur leading to death.

---

[9] The ingredients of this formula are not given in this book.

Formulas for the Treatment of Injury Due to *Dian Xue* or Spotting

163. Rx ... *Fan Du* (*i.e.*, *Zhang Men*, Liv 13)

Rx 1. Rx #192 plus Semen Alpiniae Katsumadai (*Cao Dou Kou*), 3g, Radix Saussureae Seu Vladimiriae (*Mu Xiang*), 3g, defatted Semen Crotonis Tiglii (*Ba Dou Shuang*), 2.4g. Decoct with water and take.

Rx 2. First take 0.9g of *Qi Li San* (7 *Li* Powder). Then take 9g of *Di Bie Zi Jin Dan* (Eupolyphaga Purple Gold Elixir). Apply locally as a poultice ingredients with a pulling property. If this injury is not cured, the case will become critical and recalcitrant to treatment.

164. Rx ... *Fu Jie* (Sp 14)

Rx 1. Rx #192 plus Semen Pruni Persicae (*Tao Ren*), 4.5g, Rhizoma Corydalis Yanhusuo (*Yan Hu Suo*), 4.5g. Decoct with water and take.

Rx 2. Nine tenths of a gram of *Qi Li San* (7 *Li* Powder) and 3 *ji* of *Duo Ming Dan* (Extend the Life Elixir).

165. Rx ... *Dan Tian*[10]

Rx #192 plus Rhizoma Sparganii (*San Leng*), 4.5g, Caulis Akebiae Mutong (*Mu Tong*), 4.5g. Decoct with water and take. This can be supplemented with 0.9g of *Qi Li San* (7 *Li* Powder) taken with yellow wine (*i.e.*, rice wine).

Note: The *dan tian* homes to the small intestine and kidney channels. If injury to this area is not cured in time, it will become recalcitrant to treatment afterward.

---

[10] The *dan tian* corresponds to the area between *Qi Hai* (CV 6) and *Guan Yuan* (CV 4).

166. Rx ... *Shui Fen* (CV 9)

Rx #192 plus Rhizoma Atractylodis Macrocephalae (*Bai Zhu*), Rhizoma Sparganii (*San Leng*), raw Radix Glycyrrhizae (*Sheng Gan Cao*), 4.5g each. Decoct with water and take. This should be taken with 0.9g of *Qi Li San* (7 *Li* Powder) and *Di Bie Zi Jin Dan* (Eupolyphaga Purple Gold Elixir).

Commentary: This point homes to the bladder channel. It is the intersection point of the qi of both the large and small intestine channels. If it is spotted, obstruction of urination and defecation may occur. If not cured in time, such injury will be recalcitrant to treatment afterward.

167. Rx ... *Qi Ge*

Rx #192 plus Cortex Radicis Acanthopanacis (*Wu Jia Pi*), Radix Et Rhizoma Notopterygii (*Qiang Huo*), 4.5g each. Decoct with water and take. Then take 0.7g of *Qi Li San* (7 *Li* Powder) and 3 *ji* of *Duo Ming Dan* (Extend the Life Elixir).

Commentary: If this point is spotted, treat immediately. Otherwise such injury will be difficult to cure.

Note: *Qi Ge* is located 5 *fen* lateral to *Ge Shu*.

168. Rx ... *Guan Yuan* (CV 4)

Rx #192 plus Pericarpium Viridis Citri Reticulatae (*Qing Pi*), Semen Plantaginis (*Che Qian Zi*), 6g each. Decoct with water and take. This can be supplemented with 0.9g of *Qi Li San* (7 *Li* Powder) and 3 *ji* of *Duo Ming Dan* (Extend the Life Elixir).

Formulas for the Treatment of Injury Due to *Dian Xue* or Spotting

Commentary: This point can be interpreted as the *dan tian*. It is the source from which the qi effuses during martial training. If injured, treat immediately to prevent further deterioration.

169. Rx ... *Xue Hai Men*

Rx #192 plus Radix Bupleuri (*Chai Hu*), 4.5g, Radix Angelicae Sinensis (*Dang Gui*), 4.5g. Decoct with water and take. Add 0.7g of *Qi Li San* (7 *Li* Powder) taken with yellow wine (*i.e.*, rice wine). Then take 3 *ji* of *Duo Ming Dan* (Extend the Life Elixir).

Note: *Xue Hai Men* is located 2 *cun* below the left nipple.

170. Rx ... *Qi Ge Men*

Rx #192 plus Cortex Magnoliae Officinalis (*Hou Po*), Feces Trogopterori Seu Pteromi (*Wu Ling Zhi*), Fructus Amomi (*Sha Ren*), 3g each. Decoct with water and take. Then take 3 *ji* of *Duo Ming Dan* (Extend the Life Elixir).

Note: *Qi Ge Men* is located 2 *cun* below the right nipple.

171. Rx ... *Xue Nang*

Rx #192 plus Radix Angelicae Sinensis tails (*Gui Wei*), 4.5g, Lignum Sappanis (*Su Mu*), 4.5g. Decoct with water and take. Then take *Di Bie Zi Jin Dan* (Eupolyphaga Purple Gold Elixir), 4-5 doses.

Note: *Xue Nang* is located 3 *cun* below the left nipple.

172. Rx ... Wei Cang[11]

Rx #192 plus Cortex Radicis Moutan (*Dan Pi*), Flos Carthami Tinctorii (*Hong Hua*), 4.5g each. Decoct with water and take. Follow this with 3 *ji* of *Duo Ming Dan* (Extend the Life Elixir).

173. Rx ... Mei Xin (i.e., Yin Tang, EX-HN3)

Rx #192 plus Radix Ledebouriellae Sesloidis (*Fang Feng*), Radix Et Rhizoma Notopterygii (*Qiang Huo*), Herba Seu Flos Schizonepetae Tenuifoliae (*Jing Jie Sui*), Rhizoma Ligustici Wallichii (*Chuan Xiong*), 4.5g each. Decoct with water and take. Or take 0.9g of *Qi Li San* (7 *Li* Powder) and 3 *ji* of *Duo Ming Dan* (Extend the Life Elixir).

Commentary: Injury to this point is relatively easy to cure if there is an open wound, bleeding, and no swelling. If there is internal injury with swelling of the eyes and bleeding, such an injury may be difficult to cure.

174. Rx ... Qi Men (Liv 14)

Rx #192 plus Radix Albus Paeoniae Lactiflorae (*Bai Shao*), 9g, Fructus Citri Seu Ponciri (*Zhi Qiao*), Radix Bupleuri (*Chai Hu*), 4.5g each. Decoct with water and take. Follow this with 0.9g of *Qi Li San* (7 *Li* Powder) and 3 *ji* of *Duo Ming Dan* (Extend the Life Elixir).

---

[11] Point not identified.

Formulas for the Treatment of Injury Due to *Dian Xue* or Spotting

175. Rx ... *Zheng E*[12]

Rx #192 plus Radix Et Rhizoma Notopterygii (*Qiang Huo*), Radix Ledebouriellae Sesloidis (*Fang Feng*), Rhizoma Ligustici Wallichii (*Chuan Xiong*), 4.5g each. Decoct with water and take. Follow this with 3 *ji* of *Duo Ming Dan* (Extend the Life Elixir).

176. Rx ... *Xue Nang He*

Rx #192 plus Pollen Typhae (*Pu Huang*, take separately), 4.5g, powdered Semen Allii Tuberosi (*Jiu Cai Zi*, take separately), 4.5g. Follow this with 4-5 *ji* of *Duo Ming Dan* (Extend the Life Elixir).

Commentary: If 3-5 *ji* of the above still cannot relieve the occipital headache or pain and soreness of the whole body persists, the case may be difficult to cure.

Note: *Xue Nang He* is located 5 *fen* beneath the left nipple.

177. Rx ... *Da Chang Shu* (Bl 25)

Rx #192 plus Rhizoma Cyperi Rotundi (*Xiang Fu*), Fructus Citri Seu Ponciri (*Zhi Qiao*), 4.5g each, Fructus Crataegi (*Shan Zha*), 9g. Decoct with water and take. Follow this with 0.7g of *Qi Li San* (7 *Li* Powder) and 3 *ji* of *Duo Ming Dan* (Extend the Life Elixir).

178. Rx ... *Ming Men* (GV 4)

Rx #192 plus Rhizoma Ligustici Wallichii (*Chuan Xiong*), Radix Et Rhizoma Notopterygii (*Qiang Huo*), 3g. Decoct with water and take. Then take 0.6g of *Qi Li San* (7 *Li* Powder) followed by 2 *ji* of *Duo*

---

[12] Point not identified.

Ming Dan (Extend the Life Elixir). Externally powdered *Ba Bao Dan* (Eight Treasures Elixir) may be applied to the injured area.

179. Rx ... *Chang Xue* (i.e., *Gan Shu*, Bl 18)

Rx #192 plus Radix Angelicae Sinensis (*Dang Gui*), 3g, Radix Rehmanniae (*Sheng Di*), 6g, Rhizoma Ligustici Wallichii (*Chuan Xiong*), 6g. Decoct with water and take. The above ingredients should be followed by 0.6g of *Qi Li San* (7 *Li* Powder) and 3 *ji* of *Duo Ming Dan* (Extend the Life Elixir). Externally apply *Tao Hua San* (Peach Flower Powder).

180. Rx ... *Xue Zhu* (Aorta), *Zhu Ming* (i.e., *Ren Zhong*, GV 26), *Zan Ming* (i.e., *Feng Fu*, GV 16), *Hei Fu Tao Xing* (i.e., *Zhong Wan*, CV 12), *Gui Yin* (i.e., *Tian Tu*, CV 22), *You Hun* (i.e., *Tong Tian*, Bl 7)

The above 6 points are all fatal areas. If spotted, mild cases can be cured with 5-7 *ji* of Rx #192 with additions and subtractions. This should be followed by 1-3g of *Qi Li San* (7 *Li* Powder) 2 times per day taken with yellow wine (*i.e.*, rice wine). Then supplement this with 5 *ji* of *Di Bie Zi Jin Dan* (Eupolyphaga Purple Gold Elixir).

If the ribs are broken or badly injured, the use of *Shao Lin Tong Shen Gao* (Shaolin Child Birth Plaster), also known as *He Gu Yin* (Acclaimed Bone Leader), is essential. Take Semen Oryzae Glutinosae (*Nuo Mi*, 120g if fresh, 60g if old), germinate, and fry until carbonized. Then take 60g of Folium Euphorbiae Lathyridis (*Xu Sui Zi Ye*) and process with infant's urine 7 times (remove the thorns). Mix this with the ash from the rice sprouts and add 30g of Semen Levis Tritici (*Fu Xiao Mai*) and smash into a paste. Add some old vinegar (*Chen Cu*) and mix this into the paste. Then apply this paste to the affected area. Take 0.3-0.6g of *Qi Li San* (7 *Li* Powder) with yellow wine (*i.e.*, rice wine). Follow this with 3g of *Di Bie Zi*

Formulas for the Treatment of Injury Due to *Dian Xue* or Spotting

Jin Dan (Eupolyphaga Purple Gold Elixir) and 3 *ji* of *Duo Ming Dan* (Extend the Life Elixir). One may also add the ingredients of Rx #192.

181. Rx ... Various Points on the Back

Rx # 192 plus Fructus Psoraleae Corylifoliae (*Bu Gu Zhi*), Cortex Eucommiae Ulmoidis (*Du Zhong*), 6g each. Decoct with water and take. Follow this with 3 *ji* of *Duo Ming Dan* (Extend the Life Elixir).

182. Rx ... *Hai Di* (i.e., *Pang Guang Shu*, Bl 28)

Rx #192 plus Fructus Psoraleae Corylifoliae (*Bu Gu Zhi*), 4.5g, Radix Linderae Strychnifoliae (*Wu Yao*), 6g. Decoct with water and take. Follow this with 3 *ji* of *Zi Jin Dan* (Purple Gold Elixir).

183. Rx ... *Yao Yan* (EX-B7)

Rx #192 plus Semen Pruni Persicae (*Tao Ren*), Semen Euphorbiae Lathyridis (*Xu Sui Zi*), 4.5g each. Decoct with water and take. Follow this with 3 *ji* of *Duo Ming Dan* (Extend the Life Elixir).

Note: *Yao Yan* is located 2 fingerbreadths lateral to the second sacral bone. The left point homes to the kidneys, while the right point homes to the *Ming (Men)*. If spotted, one must cure this injury immediately. Otherwise, within a couple of days the case will become critical and recalcitrant to treatment.

184. Rx ... *Ming Men* (GV 4)

Rx #192 plus Semen Pruni Persicae (*Tao Ren*), Radix Peucedani (*Qian Hu*), 4.5g each. Decoct with water and take. Follow this with 3 *ji* of *Duo Ming Dan* (Extend the Life Elixir).

Commentary: If this treatment does not effect a cure, supplement the above prescription with Radix Salviae Miltiorrhizae (*Dan Shen*), 6g.

185.   Rx ... *Xia Hai Di* (i.e., *Qu Gu*, CV 2)

Rx #192 plus Radix Et Rhizoma Rhei (*Da Huang*), Borax (*Peng Sha*), Fructus Chaenomelis Lagenariae (*Mu Gua*), 6g each. Decoct with water and take. Follow this with 3 *ji* of *Duo Ming Dan* (Extend the Life Elixir).

186.   Rx ... *He Kou*[13]

Rx #192 plus Fructus Alpiniae Oxyphyllae (*Yi Zhi Ren*), Fructus Chaenomelis Lagenariae (*Mu Gua*), 3g each, Radix Achyranthis Bidentatae (*Niu Xi*), 4.5g. Decoct with water and take. Follow this with 3 *ji* of *Di Bie Zi Jin Dan* (Eupolyphaga Purple Gold Elixir).

187.   Rx ... *Yong Quan* (Ki 1)

Rx #192 plus Fructus Chaenomelis Lagenariae (*Mu Gua*), Radix Achyranthis Bidentatae (*Niu Xi*), 6g each. Decoct with water and take. If the kidneys are injured, Radix Pseudoginseng (*San Qi*, taken separately), 6g, and Fructus Alpiniae Oxyphyllae (*Yi Zhi Ren*), 6g, may be added.

188.   Rx ... *Jing Ming* (Bl 1)

Rx #192 plus Semen Cassiae Torae (*Cao Jue Ming*), Herba Equiseti Hiemalis (*Mu Zei Cao*), 6g each. Decoct with water and take. Add 0.9g of *Qi Li San* (7 *Li* Powder) taken with yellow wine (*i.e.*, rice wine).

---

[13]   Point not identified.

Formulas for the Treatment of Injury Due to *Dian Xue* or Spotting

189. Rx ... *Er Men* (TH 21)

Rx #192 plus Ramulus Cinnamomi (*Gui Zhi*), 4.5g, Rhizoma Coptidis Chinensis (*Huang Lian*), 1.5g. Decoct with water and take. Add 0.7g of *Qi Li San* (7 *Li* Powder) taken with yellow wine (*i.e.*, rice wine).

190. Rx ... *Nei Guan* (Per 6)

Rx #192 plus Radix Et Rhizoma Notopterygii (*Qiang Huo*), Ramulus Cinnamomi (*Gui Zhi*), 4.5g each, Radix Achyranthis Bidentatae (*Niu Xi*), 9g. Decoct with water and take. Follow this with 0.9g of *Qi Li San* (7 *Li* Powder) taken with yellow wine (*i.e.*, rice wine).

191. Rx ... *Xia Guan* (St 7)

Rx #192 plus Flos Carthami Tinctorii (*Hong Hua*), 5g, Fructus Chaenomelis Lagenariae (*Mu Gua*), 6g, Radix Angelicae (*Bai Zhi*), 4.5g. Decoct with water and take. Follow this with 3 *ji* of *Zi Jin Dan* (Purple Gold Elixir).

Chapter Eight

Shaolin Herbal Lore

192. *Dian Xue Ji Zhi Zong Fang (Shi San Wei Zhu Fang)* General Emergency Formula for Spotting (a.k.a. Thirteen Flavors Ruling Formula)

Rhizoma Ligustici Wallichii (*Chuan Xiong*), 6g, Radix Angelicae Sinensis (*Dang Gui*), 9g, Rhizoma Corydalis Yanhusuo (*Yan Hu Suo*), 6g, Radix Saussureae Seu Vladimiriae (*Mu Xiang*), 9g, Pericarpium Viridis Citri Reticulatae (*Qing Pi*), 6g, Radix Linderae Strychnifoliae (*Wu Yao*), 6g, Semen Pruni Persicae (*Tao Ren*), 6g, Radix Polygalae Tenuifoliae (*Yuan Zhi*), 6g, Rhizoma Sparganii (*San Leng*), 4.5g, Rhizoma Curcumae Zedoariae (*E Zhu*), 6g, Rhizoma Drynariae (*Gu Sui Bu*), 6g, Radix Rubrus Paeoniae Lactiflorae (*Chi Shao*), 6g, Lignum Sappanis (*Su Mu*), 6g

In case of constipation, add raw Radix Et Rhizoma Rhei (*Da Huang*), 6g. For anuria, add Semen Plantaginis (*Che Qian Zi*), 9g. For poor appetite, add Cortex Magnoliae Officinalis (*Hou Po*) and Fructus Amomi (*Sha Ren*), 6g each. Add 2 bowls of water and decoct reducing the liquid to ½ bowl. Dilute the juice and take with yellow wine (*i.e.*, rice wine).

Note: The basic ingredients number 13; hence the name.

193. Shao Lin Pai Du Tang
Shaolin Toxin-expelling Decoction

Flos Lonicerae Japonicae (*Jin Yin Hua*), Fructus Forsythiae Suspensae (*Lian Qiao*), 15g each, Herba Cum Radice Violae Yedoensis (*Di Ding*), 30g, Sichuan Rhizoma Coptidis Chinensis (*Chuan Huang Lian*), 9g, Cortex Phellodendri (*Huang Bai*), 9g, Radix Rumicis Japonici (*Yang Di Gen*), 30g, Radix Angelicae (*Bai Zhi*), 6g, Squama Manitis Pentadactylis (*Chuan Shan Jia*), 9g, Bulbus Fritillariae Thunbergii (*Zhe Bei Mu*), 9g, Rhizoma Phragmitis Communis (*Lu Gen*), 6g, Cortex Radicis Moutan (*Dan Pi*), 12g, raw Radix Glycyrrhizae (*Sheng Gan Cao*), 6g

Decoct in water and take, each day 1 *ji*. Take together with yellow wine (*i.e.*, rice wine).

194. Jia Jian Shi San Wei Fang
Modified Thirteen Flavors Formula

Radix Polygalae Tenuifoliae (*Yuan Zhi*, remove the heart), 4.5g, Herba Artimisiae Anomalae (*Liu Ji Nu*), 6g, Cortex Cinnamomi (*Rou Gui*), 4.5g, Guangdong Pericarpium Citri Reticulatae (*Guang Chen Pi*), 6g, Cortex Eucommiae Ulmoidis (*Du Zhong*), 6g, Radix Angelicae Sinensis (*Dang Gui*), 9g, Rhizoma Corydalis Yanhusuo (*Yan Hu Suo*), 6g, Fructus Amomi (*Sha Ren*), 6g, Cortex Radicis Acanthopanacis (*Wu Jia Pi*), 9g, Feces Trogopterori Seu Pteromi (*Wu Ling Zhi*), 6g, raw Pollen Typhae (*Sheng Pu Huang*), 6g, Fructus Citri Seu Ponciri (*Zhi Qiao*), 4.5g, Herba Lycopi Lucidi (*Ze Lan*), 9g

Decoct in water and take.

Functions: Breaks stasis and engenders new (tissue), quickens the blood and rectifies the qi, disperses swelling and scatters nodulation, supplements the kidneys and strengthens the low back

This formula can be used in all cases of redness, swelling, pain due to blood stasis accumulation and gathering, fracture, dislocation, lumbago, and pain in the eyes due to fall and strike and external injury.

Commentary: This formula was created by a famous monk called Fu Yu who was given a title by the emperor of the Song Dynasty. He based this formula on his scores of years of clinical experience. It is efficacious in the treatment of all kinds of contusions and injuries.

195. *Shao Lin Si Mi Chuan Yao An* Shaolin Monastery Secret Transmission Herbal Lore

Radix Angelicae Sinensis tails (*Gui Wei*), Rhizoma Ligustici Wallichii (*Chuan Xiong*), Radix Rehmanniae (*Sheng Di*), Radix Dipsaci (*Chuan Duan*), 6g each, Lignum Sappanis (*Su Mu*), Gummum Olibani (*Ru Xiang*, remove the oil), Myrrha (*Mo Yao*, remove the oil), Caulis Akebiae Mutong (*Mu Tong*), Radix Linderae Strychnifoliae (*Wu Yao*), Herba Lycopi Lucidi (*Ze Lan*), 3g each, Semen Pruni Persicae (*Tao Ren*, remove the skin & tip), 14 kernels, Radix Glycyrrhizae (*Gan Cao*), 2.4g, Radix Saussureae Seu Vladimiriae (*Mu Xiang*), 2.1g, raw Rhizoma Zingiberis (*Sheng Jiang*), 3 slices

Decoct in water, add infant's urine and also 1 cup of wine, and take internally.

Commentary: This formula was created by the great Shaolin monk Hen Ling who was a master of martial arts of the Qing Dynasty and a hermit monk of Fen Deng County, Hui Ke, on the basis of their each 50 years' clinical experience. It has been proven efficacious in the treatment of fractures and dislocation due to fighting.

196. Fa San Shang Bu Fang
Rx for Effusing & Scattering the Upper Part

When a person is injured in their upper, middle, and lower parts, the treatment needs to first take 1-2 *ji* of ingredients with effusing and scattering properties so that the toxins can be resolved and expelled through perspiration. This will speed the recovery.

Radix Ledebouriellae Sesloidis (*Fang Feng*), Rhizoma Ligustici Wallichii (*Chuan Xiong*), Radix Angelicae Sinensis tails (*Gui Wei*), Radix Rubrus Paeoniae Lactiflorae (*Chi Shao*), Pericarpium Citri Reticulatae (*Chen Pi*), Radix Et Rhizoma Notopterygii (*Qiang Huo*), processed Rhizoma Pinelliae Ternatae (*Ban Xia*), 6g each, Radix Angelicae (*Bai Zhi*), Guangdong Radix Saussureae Seu Vladimiriae (*Guang Mu Xiang*), Radix Glycyrrhizae (*Gan Cao*), 3g each, Radix Angelicae Pubescentis (*Du Huo*), Rhizoma Drynariae (*Gu Sui Bu*), 4.5g each, raw Rhizoma Zingiberis (*Sheng Jiang*), 3 slices

Decoct in equal parts water and wine and take.

Commentary: This formula is used mainly for injuries of the face, head, neck, and upper limbs.

197. Fa San Zhong Bu Fang
Rx for Effusing & Scattering the Middle Part

Cortex Eucommiae Ulmoidis (*Du Zhong*), Radix Dipsaci (*Chuan Xu Duan*), Bulbus Fritillariae (*Bei Mu*), Semen Pruni Persicae (*Tao Ren*), Herba Artimisiae Anomalae (*Liu ji Nu*), Fructus Viticis (*Man Jing Zi*), 6g each, Radix Angelicae Sinensis (*Dang Gui*), Radix Rubrus Paeoniae Lactiflorae (*Chi Shao*), Pyritum (*Zi Ran Tong*, dipped in vinegar 7 times), 9g each, Cortex Cinnamomi (*Rou Gui*), 2.4g, Radix Rubiae Cordifoliae (*Qian Cao*), 3g

Decoct in equal parts water and wine. To improve its therapeutic effect, add 1 spoon of ginger juice (*Jiang Zhi*) and take internally.

Commentary: This prescription is mainly for the treatment of injuries of the body trunk, chest, abdomen, and back.

198. *Fa San Xia Bu Fang*
Rx for Effusing & Scattering the Lower Part

Radix Achyranthis Bidentatae (*Niu Xi*), Fructus Chaenomelis Lagenariae (*Mu Gua*), Radix Angelicae Pubescentis (*Du Huo*), 9g each, Radix Angelicae Sinensis tails (*Gui Wei*), Rhizoma Ligustici Wallichii (*Chuan Xiong*), 6g, each, Radix Dipsaci (*Chuan Duan*), Cortex Magnoliae Officinalis (*Hou Po*), Radix Clematidis Chinensis (*Wei Ling Xian*), Radix Rubrus Paeoniae Lactiflorae (*Chi Shao*), Flos Lonicerae Japonicae (*Jin Yin Hua*), 7.5g each, Radix Glycyrrhizae (*Gan Cao*), 3g

Decoct in equal parts water and wine. For better results, add 1 spoon of ginger juice (*Jiang Zhi*) and take internally.

Commentary: This prescription is mainly used for injuries of the lower extremities and private parts.

Chapter Nine

Modified Prescriptions for the Universal Treatment of Fall & Strike Injuries

199. Rx for the Treatment of Static Blood Congealed in the Chest Due to Injury

Modified 13 Flavor Rx plus Fructus Cardamomi (*Kou Ren*), 4.5g. Take with 30g of yellow wine (*i.e.*, rice wine) after being decocted with water.

200. Rx for the Treatment of Injury of the Heart Attacked by the Blood with Qi on the Verge of Exhaustion

Mod. 13 plus Semen Praeparatus Sojae (*Dan Dou Chi*), 3g. Take with 30g of yellow wine (*i.e.*, rice wine) after being decocted with water.

201. Rx ... Injury within the Heart Attacked by the Qi

Mod. 13 plus Flos Caryophylli (*Ding Xiang*), 3g. Decoct with water and take.

202. Rx ... Qi Panting Due to Injury

Mod. 13 plus Semen Pruni Armeniacae (*Xing Ren*), Fructus Citri Seu Ponciri (*Zhi Qiao*), 3g each. Decoct with water and take.

203. Rx ... Raving Caused by Martial Injury

Mod. 13 plus Radix Panacis Ginseng (*Ren Shen*), 3g, Cinnabar (*Zhu Sha*, powder & take separately), 1.5g. The above medicinals should be decocted in gold and silver vessels. Drink the juice.

204. Rx ... Loss of Hearing Due to Injury

Mod. 13 plus Radix Saussureae Seu Vladimiriae (*Mu Xiang*), Rhizoma Acori Graminei (*Shi Chang Pu*), 3g each. Decoct with water and take.

205. Rx ... Qi Obstruction Due to Injury

Mod. 13 plus Cortex Magnoliae Officinalis (*Hou Po*), Radix Gentianae Scabrae (*Long Dan Cao*), 3g each, Pericarpium Citri Reticulatae (*Chen Pi*), 1.5g. Decoct with water and take.

206. Rx ... Fever Due to Injury

Mod. 13 plus Radix Scutellariae Baicalensis (*Huang Qin*), Radix Bupleuri (*Chai Hu*), Radix Albus Paeoniae Lactiflorae (*Bai Shao*), Herba Menthae (*Bo He*), Radix Ledebouriellae Sesloidis (*Fang Feng*), 3g each, Herba Cum Radice Asari (*Xi Xin*), 1.8g. Decoct with water and take.

207. Rx ... Blood Stasis Due to Injury

Mod. 13 plus Crinis Carbonisatus (*Xue Yu Tan*), 6g. First decoct with water and then add yellow wine (*i.e.*, rice wine).

208. Rx ... Mania Due to Injury

Mod. 13 plus raw Pollen Typhae (*Sheng Pu Huang*), 3g, Sichuan Rhizoma Coptidis Chinensis (*Chuan Huang Lian*), 6g. Decoct with water and take.

209. Rx ... Low Back Pain Due to Martial Injury

Mod. 13 plus Cortex Eucommiae Ulmoidis (*Du Zhong*), Fructus Psoraleae Corylifoliae (*Bu Gu Zhi*), 3g each, Cortex Cinnamomi (*Rou Gui*), Fructus Foeniculi Vulgaris (*Xiao Hui Xiang*), 2.4g each.

210. Rx ... Stools Not Free-flowing (*i.e.*, Constipation) Due to Injury

Mod. 13 plus Radix Angelicae Sinensis (*Dang Gui*), Radix Et Rhizoma Rhei (*Da Huang*), 6g each, Mirabilitum (*Mang Xiao*, take separately), 3g

211. Rx ... Urine Not Free-flowing Due to Injury

Mod. 13 plus Flos Seu Herba Schizonepetae Tenuifoliae (*Jing Jie Sui*), Radix Et Rhizoma Rhei (*Da Huang*), Herba Dianthi (*Qu Mai*), 3g each, Semen Pruni Armeniacae (*Xing Ren*, remove skin & tips), 14 kernels. Decoct with water and take.

212. Rx ... Hemafecia Due to Injury

Mod. 13 plus Sichuan Rhizoma Coptidis Chinensis (*Chuan Huang Lian*), 3g, Cacumen Biotae Orientalis (*Ce Bai Ye*), 6g, Radix Sanguisorbae (*Di Yu*), 30g. Decoct with water and take.

213. Rx ... Hematuria Due to Injury

Mod. 13 plus Pericarpium Punicae Granati (*Shi Liu Pi*), 4.5g, eggplant calyx (*Qie Geng*), 6g. Decoct with water and take.

214. Rx ... Stools & Urine Not Free-flowing Due to Injury

Mod. 13 plus Radix Et Rhizoma Rhei (*Da Huang*), Semen Pruni Armeniacae (*Xing Ren*, remove skin & tips), Cortex Cinnamomi (*Rou Gui*), 4.5g each. Decoct with water and take.

215. Rx ... Urinary Incontinence Due to Injury

Mod. 13 plus Cortex Cinnamomi (*Rou Gui*), Flos Caryophylli (*Ding Xiang*), 3g each. Decoct with water and take.

216. Rx ... Fecal Incontinence Due to Injury

Mod. 13 plus Rhizoma Cimicifugae (*Sheng Ma*), Radix Astragali Membranacei (*Huang Qi*), Fructus Terminaliae Chebulae (*He Zi*), Radix Platycodi Grandiflori (*Jie Geng*), 3g each. Decoct with water and take.

217. Rx ... Chilly Pain in the Intestines Due to Injury

Mod. 13 plus Rhizoma Corydalis Yanhusuo (*Yan Hu Suo*), Rhizoma Alpiniae Officinari (*Gao Liang Jiang*), 3g each. Decoct with water and take.

218. Rx ... Cough Due to Injury

Mod. 13 plus Gelatinum Corii Asini (*E Jiao*), 6g. After taking this decoction, take 1 cup of Herba Allii Tuberosi juice (*Jiu Cai Zhi*).

219. Rx ... Pain in the Right Lower Abdomen Due to Injury

Mod. 13 plus Fructus Amomi Tsao-ko (*Cao Guo*), Fructus Forsythiae Suspensae (*Lian Qiao*), Radix Angelicae (*Bai Zhi*), 3g each. Decoct with water and take.

220. Rx ... Hematemesis Due to Injury

Mod. 13 plus Pollen Typhae (*Pu Huang*), Rhizoma Imperatae Cylindricae (*Bai Mao Gen*), 3g each. Decoct with water and take.

221. Rx ... Bad Smell Emanating from the Mouth Due to Injury

Mod. 13 plus Flos Caryophylli (*Ding Xiang*), Fructus Amomi Tsao-ko (*Cao Guo*), processed Rhizoma Pinelliae Ternatae (*Ban Xia*), 3g each, Fructus Amomi (*Sha Ren*), 7 kernels, Semen Phaseoli Calcarati (*Chi Xiao Dou, i.e.,* aduki beans), 100 grains. Decoct with water and take.

222. Rx ... Hearing Not Clear Due to Shortening of the Tongue Due to Detriment & Damage

Mod. 13 plus Radix Panacis Ginseng (*Ren Shen*), Rhizoma Coptidis Chinensis, raw Gypsum Fibrosum (*Sheng Shi Gao*), 3g each. Decoct with water and take.

223. Rx ... Elongated Tongue Due to Injury

Mod. 13 plus fresh Bombyx Batryticatus (*Sheng Jiang Can*), Terra Flava Usta (*Fu Long Gan*), 3g each, raw iron slag (*Sheng Tie Lou*), 120g. Decoct with water and take.

224. Rx ... Hiccough Due to Injury

Mod. 13 plus Radix Bupleuri (*Chai Hu*), Cortex Radicis Acanthopanacis (*Wu Jia Pi*), Fructus Chaenomelis Lagenariae (*Mu Gua*), Semen Plantaginis (*Che Qian Zi*), 3g each. Decoct with water and take.

225. Rx ... Bleeding from the 9 Portals[1] Due to Injury

Mod. 13 plus Semen Momordicae Cochinensis (*Mu Bie Zi*), Cortex Cercis Chinensis (*Zi Jing Pi*), 3g each. Decoct in water, add 1 cup of infant's urine, and take.

226. Rx ... Difficulty in Turning Body to the Side Due to Injury

Mod. 13 plus Radix Morindae Officinalis (*Ba Ji Tian*), Cortex Eucommiae Ulmoidis (*Du Zhong*), Radix Achyranthis Bidentatae (*Niu

---

[1] Eyes, ears, both nostrils, mouth, anus & urethra

Xi), Ramulus Cinnamomi (*Gui Zhi*), 3g each. Decoct with water and take.

227. Rx ... Loss of Consciousness Due to Injury

Mod. 13 plus Radix Saussureae Seu Vladimiriae (*Mu Xiang*), Cinnabar (*Zhu Sha*, powder & take separately), Borax (*Peng Sha*, powder & take separately), Succinum (*Hu Po*, powder & take separately), 3g each, Western Radix Codonopsis Pilosulae (*Xi Dang Shen*), 15g. Decoct with water and take.

228. Rx ... Heart Attacked by Qi & Blood Due to Injury

Mod. 13 plus black chicken[2] soup (*Hei Ji Tang*). Black chicken soup's method of preparation: Kill a black chicken and wash it clean. Take out the internal organs. Put it in a clay pot. Cook with equal parts water and yellow wine (*i.e.*, rice wine). Take the soup mixed with black bean juice (*Hei Dou Zhi*).

229. Rx ... Splitting Headache Due to Injury

Mod. 13 plus Herba Cistanchis (*Rou Cong Rong*), Radix Angelicae (*Bai Zhi*), 3g each. Decoct with water and take.

---

[2] Black chickens are a particular variety raised in China with white feathers but with black skin and flesh due to unusually high amounts of melanin. Their meat is especially effective for tonifying the Blood. It is a main ingredient in the several versions of Black Chicken White Phoenix Pills, a common gynecological patent medicine.

230. Rx ... Headache at the Vertex Due to Injury

Mod. 13 plus Cortex Magnoliae Officinalis (*Hou Po*), Radix Scutellariae Baicalensis (*Huang Qin*), Radix Et Rhizoma Ligustici Sinensis (*Gao Ben*), 3g each. Decoct with water and take.

231. Rx ... Redness & Swelling of the Eyes Due to Injury

Mod. 13 plus Semen Cassiae Torae (*Cao Jue Ming*), 4.5g, Fructus Viticis (*Man Jing Zi*), 1.3g. Decoct with water and take.

232. Rx ... Nosebleed Due to Broken Nose Due to Martial Injury

Mod. 13 plus Flos Magnoliae (*Xin Yi*), Carapax Amydae Sinensis (*Bie Jia*), 3g each. Decoct with water and take.

233. Rx ... Bleeding from the Ears Due to Martial Injury

Mod. 13 plus Magnetitum (*Ci Shi*, powdered & take separately), 3g. Decoct with water and take.

234. Rx ... Injury to the Throat Due to Fighting

Mod. 13 plus green carp gallbladder (*Qing Yu Dan*), 1.5g, *Qing Liang San* (Clear Cool Powder, a patent medicine; take separately). Decoct in water and take.

235. Rx ... Cheek Injury Due to Fighting

Mod. 13 plus Radix Angelicae Pubescentis (*Du Huo*), Herba Cum Radice Asari (*Xi Xin*), 3g each. Decoct with water and take.

236. Rx ... Split Lips Due to Fighting

Mod. 13 plus Rhizoma Cimicifugae (*Sheng Ma*), Radix Gentianae Macrophyllae (*Qin Jiao*), Radix Achyranthis Bidentatae (*Niu Xi*), 3g each. Decoct with water and take.

237. Rx ... Loss of Teeth Due to Fighting

Mod. 13 plus Scapus Eriocaulonis Buergerani (*Gu Jing Cao*), 3g. Decoct with water and take.

238. Rx ... Loose Teeth Due to Fighting

Mod. 13 plus Radix Angelicae Pubescentis (*Du Huo*), 3g, Herba Cum Radice Asari (*Xi Xin*), 2.1g. Decoct with water and take. Use Galla Rhi Chinensis (*Wu Bei Zi*), Lumbricus (*Di Long*), Radix Saussureae Seu Vladimiriae (*Mu Xiang*) in equal portions. Powder, make a paste, and apply to the gums.

239. Rx ... Shoulder Pain Due to Fighting

Mod. 13 plus Pericarpium Viridis Citri Reticulatae (*Qing Pi*), 4.5g. Decoct with water and take.

240. Rx ... Pain of the Arm & Hand Due to Fighting

Mod. 13 plus Ramulus Cinnamomi (*Gui Zhi*), Limonitum (*Yu Liang*), 3g each. Decoct with water, add 3 spoonfuls of ginger juice (*Jiang Zhi*), and take.

241. Rx ... Injury of the Chest Due to Fighting

Mod. 13 plus Radix Bupleuri (*Chai Hu*), Fructus Citri Seu Ponciri (*Zhi Qiao*), 3g each. Decoct with water, add 1 cup of Herba Allii Tuberosi (*Jiu Cai Zhi*) juice, and take.

242. Rx ... Injury of the Left Ribs Due to Fighting

Mod. 13 plus Semen Sinapis Albae (*Bai Jie Zi*), Radix Bupleuri (*Chai Hu*), 3g each. Decoct with water and take.

243. Rx ... Injury of the Right Ribs Due to Fighting

Mod. 13 plus Fructus Kochiae Scopariae (*Di Fu Zi*), Semen Sinapis Albae (*Bai Jie Zi*), Radix Astragali Membranacei (*Huang Qi*), 3g each, Rhizoma Cimicifugae (*Sheng Ma*), 1.5g. Decoct with water and take.

244. Rx ... Abdominal Injury Due to Fighting

Mod. 13 plus Pericarpium Arecae Catechu (*Da Fu Pi*), 3g. Decoct with water and take.

245. Rx ... Injury of the Upper Back Due to Fighting

Mod. 13 plus Radix Saussureae Seu Vladimiriae (*Mu Xiang*), Fructus Amomi (*Sha Ren*), 3g each. Decoct with water and take.

246. Rx ... Low Back Injury Due to Fighting

Mod. 13 plus Cortex Eucommiae Ulmoidis (*Du Zhong*), Fructus Psoraleae Corylifoliae (*Bu Gu Zhi*), 3g each. Decoct with water and take.

247. Rx ... Shooting Pain from the Lower to Upper Back Due to Fighting

Mod. 13 plus Semen Impatientis (*Ji Xing Zi*), 6g. Decoct with water and take.

248. Rx ... Bilateral Hip Pain Due to Fighting

Mod. 13 plus Semen Cnidii Monnieri (*She Chuang Zi*), Flos Immaturus Sophorae Japonicae (*Huai Hua*), 3g each. Decoct with water and take.

249. Rx ... Injury of Kidneys Due to Fighting

Decoct and take Rx Mod. 13. Then pulverize Secretio Moschi Moschiferi (*She Xiang*), 0.6g, Camphora (*Chang Nao*), 0.9g and mix with fresh lettuce juice (*Xian Wo Ju Zhi*) to form a paste. Apply this paste to the affected area. Instantaneous results!

250. Rx ... Anal Bleeding Due to Fighting

Mod. 13 plus stir-fried Radix Et Rhizoma Rhei (*Da Huang*), Semen Arecae Catechu (*Bing Lang*), Flos Immaturus Sophorae Japonicae (*Huai Hua*), 3g each. Decoct with water and take.

251. Rx ... Swelling & Pain of the Leg Due to Fighting

Mod. 13 plus Radix Achyranthis Bidentatae (*Niu Xi*), Herba Dendrobii (*Shi Hu*), Fructus Chaenomelis Lagenariae (*Mu Gua*), Cortex Radicis Acanthopanacis (*Wu Jia Pi*), Caulis Perillae Frutescentis (*Su Geng*), 3g each. Decoct with water and take.

252. Rx ... Heel Injury Due to Fighting

Mod. 13 plus Fructus Foeniculi Vulgaris (*Xiao Hui Xiang*), Cortex Cercis Chinensis (*Zi Jing Pi*), Lignum Sappanis (*Su Mu*), 3g each. Decoct with water and take.

253. Rx ... Joint Injury Due to Fighting

Mod. 13 plus Sclerotium Pararadix Poriae Cocos (*Fu Shen*), heartwood of Lignum Sappanis (*Su Mu Xin*), 6g each, Fructus Xanthii (*Cang Er Zi*), Rhizoma Drynariae (*Gu Sui Bu*), 3g each. Decoct with water and take.

254. Rx ... Swelling & Pain Due to Static Blood, Accumulations & Gatherings Due to Fighting

Take internally Rx Mod. 13. Also puncture with a silver needle the point *Tian Ying* which is also known as *Shang Xing* (GV 23) and the local area. This will effect a speedy cure.

255. Rx ... Fever & Poor Appetite Due to Fighting

Mod. 13 plus Pericarpium Citri Reticulatae (*Chen Pi*), 1.5g, Radix Astragali Membranacei (*Huang Qi*), Rhizoma Atractylodis Macrocephalae (*Bai Zhu*), 3g each, Rhizoma Coptidis Chinensis (*Huang Lian*), 2.4g. Decoct with water and take.

256. Rx ... Persistent Local Swelling Due to Fighting

Mod. 13 plus prepared Radix Rehmanniae (*Shu Di*), Cortex Eucommiae Ulmoidis (*Du Zhong*), Rhizoma Atractylodis (*Cang Zhu*), 6g each. Decoct with water and take.

257. Rx ... Local Bruise, Swelling & Aversion to Cold Due to Fighting

Mod. 13 plus Fructus Crataegi (*Shan Zha*), Radix Dioscoreae Oppositae (*Shan Yao*), Cortex Magnoliae Officinalis (*Hou Po*), Rhizoma Atractylodis Macrocephalae (*Bai Zhu*), Radix Bupleuri (*Chai Hu*), 3g each, Fructus Amomi (*Sha Ren*), 7 pods. Decoct with water and take.

258. Rx ... Sallow Complexion, Persistent Greenish Swelling & Alternating Fever & Chills Due to Fighting

Mod. 13 plus Radix Panacis Ginseng (*Ren Shen*), 9g, Radix Astragali Membranacei (*Huang Qi*), 30g, Rhizoma Atractylodis Macrocephalae (*Bai Zhu*), Rhizoma Cimicifugae (*Sheng Ma*), Radix Bupleuri (*Chai Hu*), 4.5g each, Pericarpium Citri Reticulatae (*Chen Pi*), 2.4g. Decoct with water and take.

259. Rx ... Paraplegia

Mod. 13 plus Ramus Loranthi Seu Visci (*Sang Ji Sheng*), 12g, Ramulus Cinnamomi (*Gui Zhi*), 3g, bear palms (*Xiong Zhang*), 1 pair. Decoct in equal parts wine and water. Make into a concentrated juice and take.

260. Rx ... Absence of Facial Lustre Due to Injury

Mod. 13 plus prepared Radix Rehmanniae (*Shu Di*), 12g, Radix Panacis Ginseng (*Ren Shen*), 6g, Placenta Hominis (*Zi He Che*), 15g, Rhizoma Atractylodis Macrocephalae (*Bai Zhu*), 12g. Grind these ingredients into a fine powder and make pills 1cm in diameter after mixing with honey. Take 1 pill each time, 2 times per day. Taking these pills consecutively for 45 days will bring about a satisfactory result.

Chapter Ten

Shaolin Training Herbal Prescriptions

261. *An Shen Jing Nao Fang*
Calm the Spirit & Tranquilize the Brain Formula

Ingredients: Sclerotium Pararadix Poriae Cocos (*Fu Shen*), 9g, Semen Alpiniae Oxyphyllae (*Yi Zhi Ren*), 9g, Margarita (*Zhen Zhu*, prepared with bean curd), 0.03g, Borax (*Peng Sha*, ground with water), 0.3g, Succinum (*Hu Po*, powdered), 0.6g, Cinnabar (*Zhu Sha*, ground with water), 0.6g, Radix Saussureae Seu Vladimiriae (*Mu Xiang*), 1.5g

Grind the above ingredients into extremely fine powder and keep in a bottle for use. Take 0.06g each time, 3 times per day with 30g of mixed water and wine.

262. *He Tiao Qi Ji Fang*
Harmonize & Regulate the Qi Mechanism Formula

Ingredients: Guangdong Radix Saussureae Seu Vladimiriae (*Guang Mu Xiang*), 1.5g, Radix Linderae Strychnifoliae (*Wu Yao*), 3g, Pericarpium Citri Reticulatae (*Chen Pi*), 4.5g, Fructus Foeniculi Vulgaris (*Xiao Hui Xiang*), 1.5g, Secretio Moschi Moschiferi (*She Xiang*), 0.06g, 3g.

Add the above ingredients to equal parts wine and water and decoct into a concentrated juice. Store this in a tightly sealed porcelain bottle. Each time take 0.1g. Add plain water and take internally after mixing thoroughly.

263. *Shao Lin Lian Gong Fang* Shaolin Training Formula

Ingredients: Sliced Cortex Elephantis (*Xiang Pi*), processed Rhizoma Pinelliae Ternatae (*Ban Xia*), processed Radix Aconiti (*Chuan Wu*), whole Radix Angelicae Sinensis (*Dang Gui*), Herba Orostachydis Fimbriati (*Wa Song*), Semen Sapindi Delavayi (*Pi Xiao*), Fructus Zanthoxyli Bungeani (*Chuan Jiao*), Cacumen Biotae Orientalis (*Ce Bai Ye*), Herba Mercurialis Leiocarpae (*Tou Gu Cao*), Herba Cum Radice Violae Yedoensis (*Zi Hua Di Ding*), sea salt (*Hai Yan*), Fructus Chaenomelis Lagenariae (*Mu Gua*), Flos Carthami Tinctorii (*Hong Hua*), 30g each, eagle claws (*Ying Zhao*), 1 pair

Method of preparation: Place the above 16 medicinals in a basin and add 3 kilograms of aged vinegar (*Chen Cu*) and 4 kilograms of spring water (*Qing Quan Shui*). Soak for 1 week and then add 120ml of white alcohol (*Bai Jiu*). Decant and keep in a tightly sealed porcelain bottle.

Method of use: Pour 250g of tincture into a basin before each practice session. Add 1 kilogram of boiling water. Rub the hand and arms in this bath for 30 minutes.

Functions: Quickens the blood and rectifies the qi, strengthens the sinews and bones

264. Shu Jin Dan
Soothing the Sinews Elixir

Ingredients: Radix Angelicae Sinensis (*Dang Gui*), 90g, Flos Carthami Tinctorii (*Hong Hua*), 90g, Radix Rubrus Paeoniae Lactiflorae (*Chi Shao*), 90g, Herba Ajugae (*Shu Jin Cao*), Fructus Chaenomelis Lagenariae (*Mu Gua*), Radix Cyathulae (*Chuan Niu Xi*), 90g each, Radix Ledebouriellae Sesloidis (*Fang Feng*), 60g, Radix Saussureae Seu Vladimiriae (*Mu Xiang*), Pericarpium Citri Reticulatae (*Chen Pi*), 30g each, Radix Angelicae (*Bai Zhi*), 60g, Semen Strychnotis (*Ma Qian Zi*, fry in oil & remove the hairs), 6g, Fructus Foeniculi Vulgaris (*Xiao Hui Xiang*), 15g

Method of preparation: Grind the above 12 ingredients into a fine powder. Mix this powder into a medium thick porridge made of yellow rice powder. Make into pills the size of Chinese parasol tree seeds. Dry before storing.

Method of administration: Take 3-4.5g each time with yellow wine (*i.e.*, rice wine).

Functions: Quickens the blood, scatters stasis, regulates and extends the three qi, namely ancestral qi, original qi, and defensive qi, soothes the sinews and disinhibits the joints, scatters stagnation and resolves depression

This formula is used mainly for low back and thigh aching and pain, injury of the sinews and joints, soreness and weakness of the four limbs, and general fatigue caused by exercise in beginners.

265. Lian Gong Jiu
Training Wine

Ingredients: Herba Lysionoti Pauciflorae (*Shi Lan Hua*), Herba Epimedii (*Yin Yang Huo*), Actinolitum (*Yang Qi Shi*), Fructus Psoraleae Corylifoliae (*Bu Gu Zhi*), Radix Pseudoginseng (*San Qi*), Radix Panacis Ginseng (*Ren Shen*), Hippocampus (*Hai Ma*), chopped snake (*She*), 15g each, Radix Albus Paeoniae Lactiflorae (*Bai Shao*), Semen Pruni Persicae (*Tao Ren*), Fructus Lycii Chinensis (*Qi Guo*), Fructus Rosae Laevigatae (*Jin Ying Zi*), Semen Cuscutae (*Tu Si Zi*), Cortex Eucommiae Ulmoidis (*Du Zhong*), 12g each, Pericarpium Viridis Citri Reticulatae (*Qing Pi*), 6g, Lignum Aquilariae Agallochae (*Chen Xiang*), 3g

Method of preparation: Place the above 16 ingredients in a porcelain jar and add 625g of best quality white alcohol (*Bai Jiu*) and a certain amount of spring water (*Qing Quan Shui*). Seal the lid with yellow earth. Shake the jar 1 time per day. After 100 days, decant the liquid.

Method of administration: Take 15-30ml before training.

Functions: Regulates and quickens the qi and blood, strengthens the sinews and bones. Taking it before training is best.

Note: *Shui She* means small lumps of pieces of snake. Therefore it is called chopped snake.

266. Lian Gong Chang Tong Qi Xue San
Unimpeded, Free-flowing Qi & Blood Training Powder

Ingredients: Radix Angelicae Sinensis (*Dang Gui*), Pericarpium Citri Reticulatae (*Chen Pi*), Radix Saussureae Seu Vladimiriae (*Mu Xiang*),

Semen Trichosanthis Kirlowii (*Lou Ren*), Radix Glycyrrhizae (*Gan Cao*) 3g each, Radix Rehmanniae (*Sheng Di*), Rhizoma Atractylodis Macrocephalae (*Bai Zhu*), Radix Astragali Membranacei (*Huang Qi*), 6g each, Radix Dioscoreae Oppositae (*Shan Yao*), 15g, Fructus Foeniculi Vulgaris (*Xiao Hui Xiang*), 1.5g, Lignum Aquilariae Agallochae (*Chen Xiang*), 0.6g

Grind all of these ingredients into a fine powder. Take 6-9g each time before training with yellow wine (*i.e.*, rice wine).

Commentary: This mixture has the functions of coursing and freeing the flow of qi and blood, regulating and extending the qi mechanism.

267. Shao Lin Yun Qi Dan
Shaolin Good Luck Elixir

Ingredients: Guangdong Radix Saussureae Seu Vladimiriae (*Guang Mu Xiang*), Fructus Amomi (*Hai Suo Sha*), Fructus Trichosanthis Kirlowii (*Quan Gua Lou*), red Lignum Dalbergiae Odoriferae (*Chi Jiang Xiang*), Radix Panacis Ginseng (*Ren Shen*), Radix Pseudoginseng (*San Qi*), Radix Astragali Membranacei (*Huang Qi*), prepared Radix Rehmanniae (*Shu Di*), Fructus Foeniculi Vulgaris (*Xiao Hui Xiang*), Radix Glycyrrhizae (*Gan Cao*), 3g each, Fructificatio Ganodermae Lucidi (*Ling Zhi*), Flos Carthami Tinctorii (*Hong Hua*), Fructus Alpiniae Oxyphyllae (*Yi Zhi Ren*), Pericarpium Citri Reticulatae (*Chen Pi*), Semen Biotae Orientalis (*Bai Zi Ren*), 6g each, whole Radix Angelicae Sinensis (*Dang Gui*), 15g

Method of preparation: Grind the above 16 ingredients into fine powder. Mix into a paste with aged vinegar (*Chen Cu*) and make pills the size of mung beans. Dry them thoroughly before storing.

Method of administration: Take 20 pills with 30ml of yellow wine (*i.e.*, rice wine) before training.

Commentary: *Yun Qi Dan* is capable of soothing and regulating the qi and blood, levelling yin and yang, and dominating the three qi. It is best to take before training.

268. *Shou Gong San*
Harvest the Training Powder

Ingredients: Lignum Aquilariae Agallochae (*Chen Xiang*), 6g, real Lignum Dalbergiae Odoriferae (*Jiang Xiang*), 3g, tender Exocarpium Citri Grandis (*Ju Hong*), 6g, stir-fried Fructus Citri Seu Ponciri (*Zhi Qiao*), 3g, Radix Angelicae Sinensis (*Dang Gui*), 9g, Flos Carthami Tinctorii (*Hong Hua*), 6g, Semen Pruni Persicae (*Tao Ren*), 3g

Method of preparation: Grind the above medicinals into a fine powder and keep in a bottle for use.

Method of administration: After each practice session, take 1-3g of this powder, which will regulate and extend the qi and blood of the entire body, which will then upbear and downbear itself.

Commentary: This formula, designed to be taken after training, has been handed down from a monk named Zhan Hua of the Qing Dynasty. However, its effect needs to be verified through practice.[1]

---

[1] Perhaps because this formula is *only* 100 years old?

Appendix

Chapter Seven: Prescriptions for the Treatment of *Dian Xue* or Spotting recommends numerous times the use of a prescription referred to as *Di Bi Zi Jin Dan* or simply as *Zi Jin Dan*. This formula is not discussed in any of the chapters on *Shang Ke* or *Die Da* translated for this book. Therefore we have taken the following description of the components and usage of this formula from *Fang Ji Xue (The Study of Formulas and Prescriptions)* compiled by Xu Ji-qun and Wang Jing-zhi, Shanghai Science & Technology Press, Shanghai, 1985:

Ingredients: Bulbus Cremastrae Seu Plieonis (*Shang Ci Gu*), 90g, Radix Knoxiae (*Jing Da Ji*), 45g, defatted Semen Euphorbiae Lathyridis (*Xu Sui Zi Shuang*), 30g, Galla Rhi Chinensis (*Wu Bei Zi*), 90g, Secretio Moschi Moschiferi (*She Xiang*), 30g, Realgar (*Xiong Huang*), 30g, Cinnabar (*Zhu Sha*), 30g

Method of Preparation: Grind the Realgar and Cinnabar with water into a fine powder. Grind the Bulbus Cremastrae, Galla Rhi Chinensis, and Radix Knoxiae also into a powder. Grind the musk seperately and then mix this with the rest of the powders. Sieve. Mix glutinous rice flour with water and knead into a lump. Steam this well and afterward mix the powdered herbs into it. Make pills and dry them in the shade.

Method of Preparation: Grind the Realgar and Cinnabar with water into a fine powder. Grind the Bulbus Cremastrae, Galla Rhi Chinensis, and Radix Knoxiae also into a powder. Grind the musk seperately and then mix this with the rest of the powders. Sieve. Mix glutinous rice flour with water and knead into a lump. Steam this well and afterward mix the powdered herbs into it. Make pills and dry them in the shade.

Dosage & administration: 0.6-1.5g per time, two times per day. For external application, regrind the pills and mix with vinegar before applying to the effected area.

Functions: Transforms phlegm and opens the portals, resolves toxins and eliminates turbidity, disperses swelling and stops pain

Indications: Accumulation of filthy, pernicious phlegm and turbidity manifesting as distention, stuffiness and pain of the gastric and abdominal area, vomiting, diarrhea, and infantile convulsions due to phlegm misting the portals. If applied externally, it treats all kinds of carbuncles, furuncles, boils, and swellings.

Index

A

abscesses, multiple 69
abdomen, and back, injuries of the body trunk, chest, 123
abdomen, pain of the lower 16, 20, 46
abdominal accumulation and lump, upper 82
abdominal injury 134
acupuncture/moxibustion 82
an mo 82
anal bleeding 135
anal prolapse 65
anesthetic 54
ankle, injury of the 83
apoplexy 65
appetite, poor 119, 136
arm, injury of the upper 83
arrow injury 30
auditory acuity, reduced 67

B

back, injury of the upper 134
back, shooting pain from the lower to upper 135
bi, wind, damp, and cold 82
Bl 1 117
Bl 12 94
Bl 13 101, 108
Bl 15 100
Bl 17 101
Bl 18 114
Bl 19 102
Bl 23 83, 93
Bl 25 113
Bl 28 115
Bl 52 96
Bl 7 114

bleeding 9-14, 22, 24, 28, 45, 87, 112, 130, 132, 135
bleeding, anal 135
bleeding due to external injury 9, 10, 45, 87
bleeding from the ears 132
bleeding from the eye 13
bleeding, localized redness, swelling, pain, and 45
blood accumulation 65, 82
blood congealed in the chest 125
blood stasis due to injury 127
blood stasis, pain due to 35, 47, 48, 53, 63, 75, 76, 82, 121
body, pain all over the 51
body, rigidity of the limbs and 47
body trunk, chest, abdomen, and back, injuries of the 123
boils of all kinds 53, 73
boils, toxic 50, 53
bone fracture 49, 76
bone fracture, acute 55
bone, injury to the 31
bruise & swelling 18
bruises 15, 42
burning and itching sensations 80

C

carbuncle on the back of the neck 69
carbuncles 40, 50, 69, 71-73, 77, 146
cheek injury 132
chest, abdomen, and back, injuries of the body trunk 123
chest, blood congealed in the 125
chest, injury of the 134
chest oppression 3
chest pain 19, 82
chest pain, side of the 82
cold accumulation 65

147

cold, aversion to 51, 137
cold limbs 65
coma 7, 65, 105
complexion, sallow 67, 137
complexion, sallow facial 43
consciousness, blurring of 2
constipation 119, 127
contusion and hit, injury due to 37
convulsions 4, 8, 49, 146
convulsions, infantile 8, 146
cough due to injury 129
CV 10 101
CV 12 82, 114
CV 15 99
CV 17 82, 102
CV 2 116
CV 21 98
CV 22 114
CV 4 109, 110
CV 6 83, 106, 109
CV 9 110

D

De Chan 3, 8, 35, 39, 40, 49, 50, 52, 71, 72, 76, 83
diarrhea 146
discharge of pus 26
disease, protracted 44
dislocation 17, 60, 75, 76, 121
dislocation of the jaw 17
dizziness 25, 41, 43, 44, 65, 67, 84
dizziness and vertigo 41, 84
dizziness, post injury hemorrhagic 25

E

ears, bleeding from the 132
ecchymosis, subdermal 49
emaciation 43, 67

eye, bleeding from the 13
eyes, deviation of the mouth and 4, 82
eyes, pain in the 121
eyes, redness & swelling of the 132

F

face, injuries of the 122
facial lustre, absence of 137
fainting due to injury 5
fatigue 43, 63, 141
fatigue caused by exercise 141
fecal incontinence 128
feet, rigidity of the hands and 75
fever 51, 126, 136, 137
fever & chills, alternating 137
fever due to injury 126
fist, injury by 18, 23
food stagnation 65
foot, injury of the dorsum of the 83
fracture and dislocation 60
fright inversion 6
Fu Hu 88
Fu Yu 39, 67, 121
furuncles 40, 50, 146

G

ganglion cysts 69
gangrene 71-73, 77
GB 20 84, 93
GB 24 106
GB 34 90
GV 16 114
GV 20 5, 84, 95
Gv 24 94
GV 26 114
GV 4 83, 91, 113, 116

Index

H

hair, premature greying of the moustache and 67
hands and feet, rigidity of the 75
head, injury to the 19, 26, 43
headache 19, 21, 51, 85, 113, 131, 132
headache at the vertex 132
headache of the forehead 21
headache, splitting 131
hearing, loss of 126
hearing not clear 130
heart, injury of the 125
heel injury 136
hemafecia 12, 88, 128
hematemesis 4, 6, 129
hematuria 11, 88, 128
hemiplegia 39, 61-63, 65, 75, 82
hemorrhage 11, 14, 24, 28, 87, 106
hemorrhagic dizziness, post injury 25
hiccough 130
hiccup 3, 98
hip pain 83, 135
hip pain, bilateral 135
Ht 7 91
Hui Ke 121

I

incontinence, fecal 128
incontinence, urinary 128
injuries of the body trunk, chest, abdomen, and back 123
injuries of the face 122
injuries of the lower extremities and private parts 123
injury by fist 18, 23
injury due to contusion and hit 37
injury due to fall 2, 23, 47, 49, 50, 57, 61-63, 76, 83
injury of the ankle 83
injury of the chest 134
injury of the dorsum of the foot 83
injury of the heart 125
injury of the left ribs 134
injury of the nose 11
injury of the right ribs 134
injury of the sinews and bones 47
injury of the sinews and joints 141
injury of the upper arm 83
injury of the upper back 134
injury of the wrist 83
injury to the bone 31
injury to the head 19, 26, 43
injury to the instep 30
injury to the neck 28
injury to the sinews 16, 18, 39, 41
injury to the throat 132
insect bites 71, 79, 80
insect bites, poisonous 71
insidious pain of the chest 15
instep, injury to the 30
intestines, chilly pain in the 129
itching 11, 31, 72, 79, 80, 82
itching sensations, burning and 80

J, K

jaw, dislocation of the 17
Ji Xue 20, 46, 61, 64, 65, 74, 80, 145
joint injury 136
joints, impeded movement of the 65
joints, inhibition of the 82
joints, injury of the sinews and 141
Ki 1 116
Ki 21 102
Ki 27 99
Ki 9 92

149

L

lateral costal area, pain in the right 22
lateral costal pain 82
leg, swelling & pain of the 135
legs, cold feeling in the 49
LI 15 83, 97
limbs and body, paralysis of the 49
limbs and body, rigidity of the 47
limbs, flaccid 43
limbs, numbness of the four 39, 61-63, 75, 82
limbs, rigidity of the four 44, 48, 51
limbs, soreness and weakness of the four 141
limbs, spastic 82
limbs, weakness of the four 65, 67, 141
lips, split 133
listlessness 85
Liv 13 100, 109
Liv 14 89, 112
localized redness, swelling, pain, and bleeding 45
lockjaw 3, 49, 89
low back and thigh aching and pain 141
low back injury 134
low back pain 20, 83, 127
low back strain 82
lower abdominal accumulation and lump 83
lower extremities and private parts, injuries of the 123
Lu 9 97
lumbar area, sprain of the 76
lumbar region and legs, soreness and pain of the 51
lumbar region, *shan* pain of the 82
lumbar sprain 60, 76

lumbosacral pain 83

M

M-HN-3 96
mania 127
martial injury 27, 126, 127, 132
mastitis 72
metal injury 10, 33
mouth, bad smell emanating from the 129
mouth, dry 3
movement, difficult 47

N

nausea 3
neck, carbuncle on the back of the 69
neck hit by fist 27
neck, injury to the 28
nose bleed 11, 132
nose, broken 132
nose, injury of the 11
nose, stuffy 51
numbness & paralysis of the lower limbs 83
numbness & paralysis of the upper limbs 83
numbness of the four limbs 39, 61-63, 75, 82

O, P

oral sores 3
osteomyelitis, suppurative 69
pain all over the body 51
pain due to blood stasis 35, 47, 48, 53, 63, 75, 76, 82, 121
pain due to unaccountable swelling 77
pain in the eyes 121

Index

pain in the right lateral costal area 22
pain in the waist and thighs 61, 62
pain, incessant 17
pain of the arm & hand 133
pain of the lower abdomen 16, 20, 46
pain of the lumbar region and thighs 41, 82
pain of the precordium 19
pallor 65
palpitations 65, 67
panting 126
paralysis 8, 49, 61, 65, 83
paralysis of the limbs and body 49
paraplegia 137
Per 6 83, 97, 117
Per 7 99
precordium, pain of the 19
prolapse of central qi 65
pus, discharge of 26

Q, R

qi accumulation 65, 82
qi inversion 2, 6, 7, 27
qi obstruction 126
ribs, injury of the left 134
ribs, injury of the right 134

S

scalding injury 83
scrofula 69
shan pain of the lumbar region 82
shoulder pain 133
shoulder, swelling & pain of the 21
shovel injury 31
SI 11 103
sinews and bones, injury of the 47
sinews, injury to the 16, 18, 39, 41
skin lesions, erosion of toxic 50

skin lesions, pernicious 25, 27, 40, 43, 53, 69, 70
skin lesions, ruptured or unruptured pernicious 53
skin rupture 24, 30
skin toxins, ulcerous 14
sores, oral 3
Sp 10 90, 106, 107
Sp 14 109
spasm 48
spear wound 10
spotting 89, 119, 145
sprain 48, 60, 76
sprain of the lumbar area 76
St 7 117
stools, loose 65
strength of the entire body, lack of 63
summerheat stroke 3, 7, 85
summerheat stroke, vertigo due to 85
suppurative conditions 33, 52
surgical treatment 54
swelling & pain of the leg 135
swelling & pain of the nape of the neck 20
swelling, pain, and bleeding, localized redness, 45
swelling, pain due to unaccountable 77
swelling, persistent greenish 137
swelling, persistent local 136

T

teeth, loose 67, 133
teeth, loss of 133
testes 92
tetanus 49
TH 21 117
thigh aching and pain, low back and 141
thighs, pain in the waist and 61, 62

151

throat, injury to the 132
throat, swelling and pain of the 3
tinnitus 67
tissue, failure to generate new 25
tongue, elongated 130
tongue, parched 3
tongue, shortening of the 130
tremor 49, 82
trismus 44, 49
tui na 82
twitching and tremor 82

U

ulcer, deeply rooted 79
ulcerated wounds 4
ulcerous lesions 24, 47, 56
ulcerous skin toxins 14
ulcers producing serous fluid 52
unconsciousness 27, 49
urinary incontinence 128
urination, clear, prolonged 65
urine not free-flowing 127, 128

V, W

vertigo due to summerheat stroke 85
vision, blurring of 43
vomiting 3, 4, 8, 98, 146
waist and thighs, pain in the 61, 62
walking, difficulty 44, 75
weakness due to protracted illness 65
weakness of the four limbs 65, 67, 141
wind, damp, and cold *bi* 82
wound, cyanotic 52
wounds due to metal weapons 45, 71
wounds, necrotic 79
wounds, suppurative and ulcerous 45
wounds, ulcerated 4
wrist, injury of the 83

X, Y, Z

Xiao Shan 83
Zhan Hua 144
Zhen Jun 3, 71, 75, 78
Zhen Zhu 48, 56, 73, 77, 88, 139

OTHER BOOKS ON CHINESE MEDICINE AVAILABLE FROM BLUE POPPY PRESS

1775 Linden Ave ○ Boulder, CO 80304
For ordering 1-800-487-9296
PH. 303\447-8372 FAX 303\447-0740

THE HEART & ESSENCE Of Dan-xi's Methods of Treatment by Zhu Dan-xi, trans. by Yang Shou-zhong. ISBN 0-936185-50-3, $24.95

HOW TO WRITE A TCM HERBAL FORMULA A Logical Methodology for the Formulation & Administration of Chinese Herbal Medicine in Decoction, by Bob Flaws, ISBN 0-936185-49-X, $10.95

FULFILLING THE ESSENCE: A Handbook of Traditional & Contemporary Chinese Treatments for Female Infertility by Bob Flaws. ISBN 0-936185-48-1, $19.95

STATEMENTS OF FACT IN TRADITIONAL CHINESE MEDICINE by Bob Flaws. ISBN 0-936185-52-X, $10.95

IMPERIAL SECRETS OF HEALTH & LONGEVITY by Bob Flaws, ISBN 0-936185-51-1, $9.95

THE MEDICAL I CHING: Oracle of the Healer Within by Miki Shima, OMD, ISBN 0-936185-38-4, $19.95

THE SYSTEMATIC CLASSIC OF ACUPUNCTURE /MOXIBUSTION by Huang-fu Mi, trans. by Yang Shou-zhong and Charles Chace, ISBN 0-936185-29-5, hardback edition, $79.95

CHINESE PEDIATRIC MASSAGE THERAPY A Parent's & Practitioner's Guide to the Treatment and Prevention of Childhood Disease, by Fan Ya-li. ISBN 0-936185-54-6, $12.95

RECENT TCM RESEARCH FROM CHINA trans. by Bob Flaws & Charles Chace. ISBN 0-936185-56-2, $18.95

PMS: Its Cause, Diagnosis & Treatment According to Traditional Chinese Medicine by Bob Flaws ISBN 0-936185-22-8 $16.95

EXTRA TREATISES BASED ON INVESTIGATION & INQUIRY: A Translation of Zhu Dan-xi's *Ge Zhi Yu Lun*, trans. by Yang Shou-zhong & Duan Wu-jin, ISBN 0-936185-53-8, $15.95

THE DIVINELY RESPONDING CLASSIC: A Translation of the *Shen Ying Jing* by Yang Shou-zhong and Liu Feng-ting, ISBN 0-936185-55-4, $18.95

A NEW AMERICAN ACUPUNCTURE: Acupuncture Osteopathy, by Mark Seem, ISBN 0-936185-44-9, $19.95

SCATOLOGY & THE GATE OF LIFE: The Role of the Large Intestine in Immunity, An Integrated Chinese-Western Approach by Bob Flaws ISBN 0-936185-20-1 $14.95

MENOPAUSE, A Second Spring: Making A Smooth Transition with Traditional Chinese Medicine by Honora Lee Wolfe ISBN 0-936185-18-X $14.95

MIGRAINES & TRADITIONAL CHINESE MEDICINE: A Layperson's Guide by Bob Flaws ISBN 0-936185-15-5 $11.95

STICKING TO THE POINT: A Rational Methodology for the Step by Step Administration of an Acupuncture Treatment by Bob Flaws ISBN 0-936185-17-1 $16.95

ENDOMETRIOSIS & INFERTILITY AND TRADITIONAL CHINESE MEDICINE: A Laywoman's Guide by Bob Flaws ISBN 0-936185-14-7 $9.95

THE BREAST CONNECTION: A Laywoman's Guide to the Treatment of Breast Disease by Chinese Medicine by Honora Lee Wolfe ISBN 0-936185-61-9 $9.95

NINE OUNCES: A Nine Part Program For The Prevention of AIDS in HIV Positive Persons by Bob Flaws ISBN 0-936185-12-0 $9.95

THE TREATMENT OF CANCER BY INTEGRATED CHINESE-WESTERN MEDICINE by Zhang Dai-zhao, trans. by Zhang Ting-liang ISBN 0-936185-11-2 $18.95

A HANDBOOK OF TRADITIONAL CHINESE DERMATOLOGY by Liang Jian-hui, trans. by Zhang Ting-liang & Bob Flaws, ISBN 0-936185-07-4 $15.95

A HANDBOOK OF TRADITIONAL CHINESE GYNECOLOGY by Zhejiang College of TCM, trans. by Zhang Ting-liang, ISBN 0-936185-06-6 (2nd edit.) $21.95

PRINCE WEN HUI'S COOK: Chinese Dietary Therapy by Bob Flaws & Honora Lee Wolfe, ISBN 0-912111-05-4, $12.95 (Published by Paradigm Press, Brookline, MA)

THE DAO OF INCREASING LONGEVITY AND CONSERVING ONE'S LIFE by Anna Lin & Bob Flaws, ISBN 0-936185-24-4 $16.95

FIRE IN THE VALLEY: The TCM Diagnosis and Treatment of Vaginal Diseases by Bob Flaws ISBN 0-936185-25-2 $16.95

HIGHLIGHTS OF ANCIENT ACUPUNCTURE PRESCRIPTIONS trans. by Honora Lee Wolfe & Rose Crescenz ISBN 0-936185-23-6 $14.95

ARISAL OF THE CLEAR: A Simple Guide to Healthy Eating According to Traditional Chinese Medicine by Bob Flaws, ISBN #-936185-27-9 $8.95

PEDIATRIC BRONCHITIS: ITS CAUSE, DIAGNOSIS & TREATMENT ACCORDING TO TRADITIONAL CHINESE MEDICINE trans. by Gao Yu-li and Bob Flaws, ISBN 0-936185-26-0 $15.95

AIDS & ITS TREATMENT ACCORDING TO TRADITIONAL CHINESE MEDICINE by Huang Bing-shan, trans. by Fu-Di & Bob Flaws, ISBN 0-936185-28-7 $24.95

ACUTE ABDOMINAL SYNDROMES: Their Diagnosis & Treatment by Combined Chinese-Western Medicine by Alon Marcus, ISBN 0-936185-31-7 $16.95

MY SISTER, THE MOON: The Diagnosis & Treatment of Menstrual Diseases by Traditional Chinese Medicine by Bob Flaws, ISBN 0-936185-34-1, $24.95

FU QING-ZHU'S GYNECOLOGY trans. by Yang Shou-zhong and Liu Da-wei, ISBN 0-936185-35-X, $21.95

FLESHING OUT THE BONES: The Importance of Case Histories in Chinese Medicine by Charles Chace. ISBN 0-936185-30-9, $18.95

CLASSICAL MOXIBUSTION SKILLS IN CONTEMPORARY CLINICAL PRACTICE by Sung Baek, ISBN 0-936185-16-3 $10.95

MASTER TONG'S ACUPUNCTURE: An Ancient Lineage for Modern Practice, trans. and commentary by Miriam Lee, OMD, ISBN 0-936185-37-6, $19.95

A HANDBOOK OF TCM UROLOGY & MALE SEXUAL DYSFUNCTION by Anna Lin, OMD, ISBN 0-936185-36-8, $16.95

Li Dong-yuan's TREATISE ON THE SPLEEN & STOMACH, A Translation of the *Pi Wei Lun* by Yang Shou-zhong & Li Jian-yong, ISBN 0-936185-41-4, $21.95

PATH OF PREGNANCY, VOL. I, Gestational Disorders by Bob Flaws, ISBN 0-936185-39-2, $16.95

PATH OF PREGNANCY, VOL. II, Postpartum Diseases by Bob Flaws, ISBN 0-936185-42-2, $18.95

How to Have a HEALTHY PREGNANCY, HEALTHY BIRTH with Traditional Chinese Medicine by Honora Lee Wolfe, ISBN 0-936185-40-6, $9.95

MASTER HUA'S CLASSIC OF THE CENTRAL VISCERA by Hua Tuo, translated by Yang Shou-zhong, ISBN 0-936185-43-0, $21.95

SEVENTY ESSENTIAL TCM FORMULAS FOR BEGINNERS by Bob Flaws, ISBN 0-936185-59-7, $19.95

CHINESE MEDICINAL WINES & ELIXIRS by Bob Flaws, ISBN 0-936185-58-9, $18.95

PAO ZHI: An Introduction to Processing Chinese Medicinals to Enhance Their Therapeutic Effect, by Philippe Sionneau, ISBN 0-936185-62-7, $24.95

THE BOOK OF JOOK: Chinese Medicinal Porridges, An Alternative to the Typical Western Breakfast, by Bob Flaws, ISBN 0-936185-60-0, $18.95